Frye's
2500
Nursing
Bullets

NCLEX-RN

FOURTH EDITION

Charles M. Frye, RN
Director
Professional Development Systems
School of Health Sciences
Long Beach, California

Springhouse Corporation
Springhouse, Pennsylvania

STAFF

Vice President
Matthew Cahill

Clinical Director
Judith Schilling McCann, RN, MSN

Art Director
John Hubbard

Managing Editor
David Moreau

Clinical Project Manager
Beverly Tscheschlog, RN

Editors
Karen Diamond, Carol Munson

Copy Editors
Brenna Mayer (manager), Priscilla
DeWitt, Mary T. Durkin, Alisa
Guerzon, Jake Marcus-Cipolla, Jaime
Stockslager, Pamela Wingrod

Designers
Arlene Putterman (associate art
director), Donna S. Morris (project
manager)

Manufacturing
Deborah Meiris (director), Patricia K.
Dorshaw (manager), Otto Mezei
(book production manager)

Editorial Assistants
Beverly Lane, Marcia Mills, Liz
Schaeffer

Indexer
Manjit K. Sahai

The clinical procedures described and recommended in this publication are based on research and consultation with nursing, medical, and legal authorities. To the best of our knowledge, these procedures reflect currently accepted practice; nevertheless, they cannot be considered absolute and universal recommendations. For individual application, all recommendations must be considered in light of the patient's clinical condition and, before administration of new or infrequently used drugs, in light of the latest package-insert information. The author and the publisher disclaim responsibility for any adverse effects resulting directly or indirectly from the suggested procedures, from any undetected errors, or from the reader's misunderstanding of the text.

Printed in the United States of America.
RNBTS4 – D N O S A J J
02 01 00   10 9 8 7 6 5 4 3 2

℞ A member of the Reed Elsevier plc group

**Library of Congress
Cataloging-in-Publication Data**

Frye, Charles M.
Frye's 2500 nursing bullets NCLEX-RN /
Charles M. Frye. —4th ed.
  p. cm.
  Includes index.
  1. Nursing Examinations, questions,
etc. 2. Nursing Outlines, syllabi, etc.
I. Frye, Charles M. Frye's 2,000 nursing
bullets NCLEX-PN. II. Title. III. Title:
2,500 nursing bullets NCLEX-RN. IV.
Title: Frye's twenty-five hundred
nursing bullets NCLEX-RN.
  [DNLM: 1. Nursing Examination
Questions. WY 18.2 F948f 1999]
RT55.F787 1999
610.73'076—dc21
DNLM/DLC   99-38477
ISBN 0-87434-985-0   CIP

To my wonderful wife,
Lailani Tisbe-Frye, RN, BSN,
who has made all of my goals achievable
and every dream a reality.

Preface

I remember in great detail preparing to take the state licensing examination for registered nurses. Of all the memories I associate with that event, the most vivid is my frantic search through the bookstores for the "right" review book that would provide answers to the test. I didn't have the time and didn't want to spend all my waking hours reading one of those 500-page review books, but nothing else was available — until now.

This book is different from other review books you've seen or used. You're holding 2,500 nursing bullets — concise information that provides answers to questions not only on the upcoming NCLEX-RN, but also on the NCLEX-PN, Commission on Graduates of Foreign Nursing Schools (CGFNS) test, and any other nursing examination. How do these bullets work for you? They're concentrated nursing facts, stated in one or two sentences that are free of unnecessary or obscure words.

Test-question writers can create lengthy and time-consuming situations, provide minute (but not necessarily meaningful) details, and ask tricky questions that any of us can misunderstand. Even so, they can't change nursing facts. These 2,500 nursing bullets are just that — facts. They're the answers you need for test questions.

Passing the examination is a necessary step in the licensing process, and you must be prepared for it. This book can help you meet that challenge. Good luck.

How to use this book

Frye's 2500 Nursing Bullets NCLEX-RN, Fourth Edition, is designed to help you review for the NCLEX-RN effectively and efficiently. This book gives you nursing information for every clinical situation and setting — the very facts that question writers must draw on in devising the test.

Follow these suggestions to get the most from this unique book:

▶ Read the introduction to prepare for computerized adaptive testing, learn about the NCLEX-RN test plan, and develop effective test-taking strategies.

▶ Study the key facts as they're presented in random order. You'll realize two benefits from this approach: You'll master essential data in psychiatric, pediatric, maternal, and medical-surgical nursing as well as the important concepts in nursing fundamentals and you'll prepare yourself for the computerized NCLEX-RN, which also presents questions in a random style. (*Note:* After each bulleted fact in this book, the applicable clinical topic area appears in parentheses: FND for fundamentals, MAT for maternal-neonatal nursing, PED for pediatric nursing, M-S for medical-surgical nursing, and PSY for psychiatric nursing.)

▶ Review groups of nursing bullets throughout the day. Because this book is compact and easy to carry, you can take it with you wherever you go and review a few bullets whenever you have a spare minute — while waiting for class to begin, during a break between labs, or while riding the bus or train.

▶ Use the book to create questions to quiz your study partner or members of your study group.

No matter how you choose to use this versatile book, you'll find that each nursing bullet is brief, easy to read, and free from distracting clinical situations and excess wording. You'll find that you'll easily remember and identify the facts, no matter what form they take on the test. Because each bullet has been reviewed by a clinical expert, you can be sure that all the information is up-to-date and clinically accurate.

You've spent years studying to become a nurse and months preparing for the NCLEX-RN. Now, with *Frye's 2500 Nursing Bullets NCLEX-RN*, Fourth Edition, you can take the last step to licensure with confidence.

Introduction

In the United States, if you want to work as a registered nurse, you need a license from the nursing licensure authority in the state where you plan to practice. To get a license, you need to pass the National Council Licensure Examination for Registered Nurses (NCLEX-RN). This book will help you do just that. Its 2,500 bullets of nursing facts will expand and reinforce your nursing knowledge base. This introduction will prepare you for the examination by describing computerized adaptive testing, explaining the NCLEX-RN test plan, and providing effective test-taking strategies.

Scheduling your test

To schedule your NCLEX-RN, apply to your state board of nursing for testing. When your application is approved, the Educational Testing Service Data Center will send you an Authorization to Test and will advise you to make an examination appointment at one of 200 Sylvan Technology Centers throughout the country.

When scheduling your NCLEX-RN, remember that the test takes up to 5 hours and is offered 15 hours daily, Monday through Saturday, and sometimes on Sunday. The Sylvan Technology Center will schedule you for testing within 30 days of your call (or within 45 days for retesting). If you need to reschedule your examination appointment, call the Sylvan Technology Center at least 3 days beforehand.

Understanding computerized adaptive testing

Since April of 1994, the NCLEX-RN has been a computerized test. It requires you to answer a sufficient number of questions of various levels of difficulty to demonstrate minimum competence as an entry-level nurse. It's adaptive because it selects harder or easier questions based on your response to previous questions. For example, if you answer a medium-level question correctly, the computer will pose a more difficult question next. If you answer incorrectly, it will choose an easier one.

The test bank includes thousands of questions categorized by level of difficulty and the NCLEX-RN test plan. From this bank, the computer continues to pull questions until you demonstrate competence in all parts of the test plan. Therefore, each test is different and may require 75 to 265 questions to complete.

Before the test, a proctor will help you get started at a computer terminal. The test will begin with brief instructions and a practice session of 15 questions. During the practice session and the test, use only the space bar (to move the cursor to the four answer options) and the enter key (to select your answer). To avoid unintentional answers, the computer will ask you to confirm your answer selection by striking the enter key again.

During the test, the computer will display one question at a time. If a case study is included, it will appear to the left of the question. Consider each question carefully. Then press the space bar to move to the option that best answers the question. To record your answer, press the enter key twice. Because the computer doesn't let you skip questions or return to previous items, you must answer every question until the test ends. The testing period includes a mandatory 10-minute break after 2 hours and an optional break 90 minutes after testing resumes.

Understanding the NCLEX-RN test plan

The NCLEX-RN test plan classifies questions by the five steps of the nursing process and the four categories of client needs. Each test question reflects one nursing process step and one client needs category.

Nursing process steps

The nursing process is a five-step method of performing nursing care. On the NCLEX-RN test, each nursing process step carries equal weight and accounts for 20% of the test questions.

▶ *Assessment* refers to forming a database by gathering subjective and objective information about a patient.

▶ *Analysis,* or nursing diagnosis, refers to identifying actual or potential health problems based on assessment findings.

▶ *Planning* refers to establishing goals to meet the patient's needs and developing strategies for achieving those goals.

▶ *Implementation* refers to performing actions that accomplish the patient's established goals.

▶ *Evaluation* refers to measuring the extent of goal achievement.

Client needs categories

Client needs categories are based on data from a major nursing job survey. These client needs are further divided into subcategories that define the content contained within each of the four major client needs categories. Each subcategory accounts for a varying percentage of the test questions.

▶ *Safe, effective care environment* refers to promoting environmental safety, providing effective care, assuring quality, and performing treatments and procedures safely and effectively. Subcategories include:

– Management of care (7% to 13% of the test)

– Safety and infection control (5% to 11% of the test).

▶ *Health promotion and maintenance* refers to meeting the patient's needs by promoting growth and development, self-care, support system integrity, and disease prevention and early treatment. Subcategories include:

– Growth and development through the life span (7% to 13% of the test)

– Prevention and early detection of disease (5% to 11% of the test).

▶ *Psychosocial integrity* refers to meeting the patient's psychosocial needs during times of stress or crisis by promoting coping skills and adaptation throughout the life cycle. Subcategories include:

– Coping and adaptation (5% to 11% of the test)

– Psychosocial adaptation (5% to 11% of the test).

▶ *Physiological integrity* refers to meeting the physiological needs of a patient with a life-threatening or recurring condition (or one at risk for complications or adverse effects of treatments) by providing care, reducing risks, and promoting physiological adaptation and comfort. Subcategories include:

– Basic care and comfort (7% to 13% of the test)

– Pharmacological and parenteral therapies (5% to 11% of the test)

– Reduction of risk potential (12% to 18% of the test)

– Physiological adaptation (12% to 18% of the test).

Studying for the examination

To study for the NCLEX-RN as effectively as possible and enhance your ability to retain pertinent information, follow these study tips:

▶ Familiarize yourself with all examination topics.

▶ Answer as many practice questions as possible. (You may want to use this book's bullets to develop questions with a study partner.)

▶ Understand the parts of a test question. On the NCLEX-RN, each multiple-choice question has a stem (the question itself) and four options: a key (correct answer) and three distracters (incorrect answers). A brief case study may precede any question.

▶ Use additional study guides as resources, such as the *American Nursing Review for NCLEX-RN*, if desired.

▶ Organize a study group with other nursing students or take an NCLEX review course.

▶ Ask a colleague or nursing instructor to clarify unfamiliar or complex material.

Planning for the examination

Remember that the NCLEX-RN poses certain physical demands. To cope with these demands, ensure your best test performance, and help you plan for the examination, use these pointers:

▶ Schedule your test appointment at a testing center near your home, if possible. Before the test, assess the parking facilities and determine travel time.

▶ Make reservations well in advance at a hotel near the testing center if you must travel a long distance.

▶ Schedule your test appointment to take advantage of your peak-performance time.

▶ Avoid late-night, last-minute cramming. Obtain sufficient sleep the night before the test.

▶ Eat a well-balanced meal before the test.

▶ Wear layers of clothes that can be removed, as needed, to maintain warmth and comfort.

▶ Take your Authorization to Test and two forms of identification with signatures (including one photographic identification) to the testing center. You can't take the examination without them.

▶ Use simple relaxation techniques, such as progressive relaxation, during the test to reduce anxiety.

Developing test-taking skills

Knowing the facts isn't all you need to pass the NCLEX-RN. You also need to know how to take the test. To sharpen your test-taking skills, review these guidelines:

▶ Check case studies closely for information needed to answer the question correctly.

▶ Look for clue words, such as *best, first, most,* and *not* in the question's stem. These words, which may be highlighted, aid in selecting the correct answer.

▶ Imagine the correct response when reading the stem. If it appears as one of the four options, it's probably the correct one.

▶ Read every question—and all four of its options—carefully before making your final selection.

▶ Reread the stem and options when two options seem equally correct; look again for clues or differences that can help you select the correct answer. When in doubt, make an educated guess. Remember: You can't skip questions.

▶ Don't panic if a question covers an unfamiliar topic. Draw on your knowledge of similar problems and nursing principles to help eliminate options and increase the chance of choosing the correct answer.

▶ Take your time and pace yourself. Don't spend excessive time on any one question.

▶ Don't be distracted by other candidates or the apparent length of their tests. Keep in mind that each test is individualized.

▶ Use break periods to rest your mind and body — for example, eat a small snack, stretch, or do relaxation exercises.

A note to foreign nurse graduates

If you were educated in a foreign country, you must meet the requirements for foreign nurse graduates set by the state board of nursing in the state where you plan to practice. Most states require a certificate from the Commission on Graduates of Foreign Nursing Schools (CGFNS) before you take the NCLEX-RN.

Eligibility requirements for the CGFNS examination include successful completion of a secondary education; a valid, current nursing license in the country in which you were educated; and graduation from a well-balanced, 2-year (or longer) nursing education program in a government-approved school.

The CGFNS examination tests your nursing knowledge and English proficiency. Its nursing portion follows the NCLEX-RN test plan and reliably predicts success on NCLEX-RN. Its English portion consists of written and listening sections. Its results reach you by mail 8 to 10 weeks after the test; passage of the test earns you a CGFNS certificate.

You can obtain application forms and the *CGFNS Guidebook for Applicants* through U.S. embassies in foreign countries, national nurses' associations, and CGFNS at 3600 Market Street, Philadelphia, PA 19104-2651. The Guidebook for Applicants presents eligibility requirements, application procedures, fees, and suggestions for CGFNS test preparation.

Frye's
2500
Nursing
Bullets

NCLEX-RN

FOURTH EDITION

▶ A child in Bryant's traction who is under age 3 or weighs less than 30 lb (13.5 kg) should have the buttocks slightly elevated and clear of the bed. The knees should be slightly flexed, and the legs should be extended at a right angle to the body. The body provides the traction mechanism. **(PED)**

▶ Unlike false labor, true labor produces regular rhythmic contractions, abdominal discomfort, no change in fetal movement, progressive fetal descent, bloody show, and progressive cervical effacement and dilation. **(MAT)**

▶ Pernicious anemia results from failure to absorb vitamin B_{12} in the GI tract and causes primarily GI and neurologic signs and symptoms. **(M-S)**

▶ In a patient with hypokalemia (serum potassium level below 3.5 mEq/L), presenting signs and symptoms include muscle weakness and cardiac arrhythmias. **(M-S)**

▶ According to Kübler-Ross, the five stages of death and dying are denial, anger, bargaining, depression, and acceptance. **(PSY)**

▶ If an I.V. route is unavailable for administering epinephrine during cardiac arrest, the medication can be administered endotracheally. **(M-S)**

▶ To help a mother break the suction of her breast-feeding infant, the nurse should teach her to insert a finger at the corner of the infant's mouth. **(MAT)**

▶ A patient with a pressure sore should consume a high-protein, high-calorie diet, unless contraindicated. **(M-S)**

▶ The creatine kinase MB-isoenzyme level is used to assess tissue damage in myocardial infarction. **(M-S)**

▶ After a 12-hour fast, the normal fasting blood glucose level ranges from 80 to 120 mg/dl. **(M-S)**

▶ A blood pressure cuff that is too narrow can cause a falsely elevated blood pressure reading. **(FND)**

▶ A blood pressure cuff that is too wide can cause a falsely decreased blood pressure reading. **(FND)**

▶ A patient with digitalis toxicity may report nausea, vomiting, diplopia, blurred vision, light flashes, and yellow-green halos around images. **(M-S)**

▶ Administering high levels of oxygen to a premature newborn can cause blindness secondary to retrolental fibroplasia. **(MAT)**

▶ When preparing a single injection for a patient who takes regular and NPH insulin, the nurse should draw the regular insulin into the syringe first because it is clear and can be measured more accurately than the NPH insulin, which is turbid. **(FND)**

▶ *Anuria* refers to a daily urine output of less than 100 ml. **(M-S)**

▶ In remittent fever, the body temperature varies over a 24-hour period but remains elevated. **(M-S)**

▶ *Rhonchi* refers to the rumbling sounds heard on lung auscultation; they are more pronounced during expiration than during inspiration. **(FND)**

▶ *Gavage* refers to forced feeding, usually through a gastric tube (a tube passed into the stomach by way of the mouth). **(FND)**

▶ Risk of a fat embolism is greatest in the first 48 hours after the fracture of a long bone and is manifested by respiratory distress. **(M-S)**

▶ To help venous blood return in a patient in shock, the nurse should elevate the patient's legs no more than 45 degrees. (This procedure is contraindicated in a patient with a head injury.) **(M-S)**

▶ According to Maslow's hierarchy of needs, physiologic needs (air, water, food, shelter, sex, activity, and comfort) have the highest priority. **(FND)**

▶ Checking the identification band on a patient's wrist is the safest and surest way to verify a patient's identity. **(FND)**

▶ A patient's safety is the priority concern in developing a therapeutic environment. **(FND)**

▶ The difference between the apical and radial pulse rates, when taken simultaneously by two nurses, is the pulse deficit. **(M-S)**

▶ The nurse should schedule postural drainage before meals or 2 to 4 hours after meals to reduce the patient's risk of vomiting and aspiration. **(M-S)**

▶ Blood pressure can be measured directly by intra-arterial insertion of a catheter connected to a pressure-monitoring device. **(M-S)**

▶ A positive Kernig's sign, seen in meningitis, occurs when an attempt to flex the hip of a recumbent patient produces painful spasms of the hamstring muscle and resistance to further leg extension at the knee. **(M-S)**

▶ In a patient with a fractured femur and displacement, treatment begins with reduction and immobilization of the affected leg. **(M-S)**

▶ Herniated nucleus pulposus (intervertebral disk) most commonly occurs in the lumbar and lumbosacral regions. **(M-S)**

▶ *Laminectomy* refers to the surgical removal of the herniated portion of an intervertebral disk. **(M-S)**

▶ Surgical treatment of a gastric ulcer includes severing the vagus nerve (vagotomy) to reduce the amount of gastric acid secreted by the gastric cells. **(M-S)**

▶ *Flight of ideas* refers to an alteration in thought processes characterized by skipping from one topic to another, unrelated topic. **(PSY)**

▶ *La belle indifference* refers to the lack of concern for a profound disability, such as blindness or paralysis, that may occur in a patient with a conversion disorder. **(PSY)**

▶ In an infant, a bulging fontanel is the most significant sign of increasing intracranial pressure. **(PED)**

▶ With moderate anxiety, a person's ability to perceive and concentrate decreases. The person is selectively inattentive (focuses on immediate concerns), and the perceptual field narrows. **(PSY)**

▶ A patient with a phobic disorder uses self-protective avoidance as the ego defense mechanism. **(PSY)**

▶ In a patient with anorexia nervosa, the highest treatment priority is correction of nutritional and electrolyte imbalances.
(PSY)

▶ A patient's blood lithium level must be monitored regularly (usually once a month) because of the narrow margin between therapeutic and toxic levels. A normal laboratory value is 0.5 to 1.5 mEq/L.
(PSY)

▶ *Valsalva's maneuver* refers to forced exhalation against a closed glottis, as when taking a deep breath, blowing air out, or bearing down.
(M-S)

▶ Early signs and symptoms of alcohol withdrawal include anxiety, anorexia, tremors, and insomnia. They may begin up to 8 hours after the last alcohol intake.
(PSY)

▶ Al-Anon is a support group for families of alcoholics. **(PSY)**

▶ The nurse shouldn't administer chlorpromazine hydrochloride (Thorazine) to a patient who has ingested alcohol because it may cause oversedation and respiratory depression. **(PSY)**

▶ Vital organ perfusion is seriously compromised when the mean arterial pressure falls below 60 mm Hg and the systolic blood pressure falls below 80 mm Hg. **(M-S)**

▶ Lidocaine hydrochloride (Xylocaine) is the drug of choice for reducing premature ventricular contractions. **(M-S)**

▶ Lithium toxicity can occur when sodium and fluid intake are insufficient, causing lithium retention. **(PSY)**

▶ *Amniotomy* refers to the artificial rupture of the amniotic membranes. **(MAT)**

▶ An alcoholic who achieves sobriety is called a *recovering alcoholic* because no cure for alcoholism exists. **(PSY)**

▶ A patient is at greatest risk of dying during the first 24 to 48 hours after a myocardial infarction. **(M-S)**

▶ The left ventricle of the heart usually sustains the greatest damage during a myocardial infarction. **(M-S)**

▶ The pain of a myocardial infarction results from myocardial ischemia caused by anoxia.   **(M-S)**

▶ For a patient in cardiac arrest, the first priority is to establish an airway.   **(M-S)**

▶ The universal sign for choking is clutching the hand to the throat.   **(M-S)**

▶ For a patient with heart failure or cardiogenic pulmonary edema, nursing interventions focus on decreasing venous return to the heart and increasing left ventricular output; these interventions include placing the patient in high Fowler's position and administering oxygen, diuretics, and positive inotropic drugs as prescribed.   **(M-S)**

▶ A positive tuberculin skin test is an induration of 10 mm or greater at the injection site.   **(M-S)**

▶ Histoplasmosis, a chronic systemic fungal infection, produces signs and symptoms that resemble those of tuberculosis. **(M-S)**

▶ Fluid oscillation in the tubing of a chest drainage system indicates that the system is working properly.   **(FND)**

▶ In burn victims, the leading cause of death is respiratory compromise; the second leading cause is infection.   **(M-S)**

▶ The exocrine function of the pancreas is the secretion of enzymes used to digest carbohydrates, fats, and proteins. **(M-S)**

▶ A patient with hepatitis A (infectious hepatitis) should consume a diet that is moderately high in fat and high in carbohydrate and protein and should eat the largest meal in the morning.   **(M-S)**

▶ The nurse should place a patient with a Sengstaken-Blakemore tube in semi-Fowler's position.   **(FND)**

▶ Esophageal balloon tamponade shouldn't be inflated greater than 20 mm Hg.   **(M-S)**

▶ Prolactin overproduction by the pituitary gland can cause galactorrhea (excessive or abnormal lactation) and amenorrhea (absence of menstruation).   **(M-S)**

▶ A classic symptom of arterial insufficiency in the leg is intermittent claudication (pain during ambulation or other movement that is relieved with rest). **(M-S)**

▶ During pregnancy, weight gain averages 25 to 30 lb (11.3 to 13.5 kg). **(MAT)**

▶ In bladder carcinoma, the most common finding is gross, painless hematuria. **(M-S)**

▶ The nurse can elicit Trousseau's sign by occluding the brachial or radial artery; hand and finger spasms during occlusion indicate Trousseau's sign and suggest hypocalcemia. **(FND)**

▶ Heparin sodium (parenteral) is contraindicated in a patient with renal or liver disease, GI bleeding, or recent surgery or trauma; in a pregnant patient; and in women over age 60. **(M-S)**

▶ Drugs that potentiate the effects of anticoagulants include aspirin, chloral hydrate, glucagon, anabolic steroids, and chloramphenicol. **(M-S)**

▶ According to Erikson, the school-age child (ages 6 to 12) is in the industry-versus-inferiority stage of psychosocial development. **(PSY)**

▶ For a burn patient, care priorities include (1) maintaining a patent airway, (2) preventing or correcting fluid and electrolyte imbalances, (3) controlling pain, and (4) preventing infection. **(M-S)**

▶ Elastic stockings should always be applied to both legs. **(M-S)**

▶ *Active immunization* refers to antibody formation within the body in response to vaccination or disease exposure. **(M-S)**

▶ *Passive immunization* refers to administration of antibodies that were preformed outside the body. **(M-S)**

▶ Chickenpox causes a rash that passes through four stages: macules, papules, vesicles, and crusts; lesions are at various stages through the illness. **(PED)**

▶ Rubella has a teratogenic effect on the fetus during the first trimester and produces abnormalities in up to 40% of cases without interrupting the pregnancy. **(MAT)**

▶ To calculate a pediatric dose using Clark's rule, the nurse should multiply the adult dose by the child's weight in pounds and divide the result by 150. **(PED)**

▶ To calculate a pediatric dose using Young's rule, the nurse should multiply the adult dose by the child's age in years and divide the result by the sum of the child's age plus 12. **(PED)**

▶ A patient receiving digoxin (Lanoxin) shouldn't receive a calcium preparation because of the increased risk of digitalis toxicity. Concomitant use may affect cardiac contractility and lead to arrhythmias. **(M-S)**

▶ For blood transfusion in an adult, the appropriate needle size is 16 to 20G. **(FND)**

▶ *Intermittent positive-pressure breathing* refers to lung inflation (during inspiration) with compressed air or oxygen under pressure from a cycling valve to keep the lung open. **(M-S)**

▶ Penicillin prophylaxis is started at age 2 months in patients with sickle cell anemia to prevent infection. **(PED)**

▶ Wristdrop results from paralysis of the extensor muscles in the forearm and hand. **(M-S)**

▶ Footdrop results from excessive plantar flexion and usually is a complication of prolonged bed rest. **(M-S)**

▶ A patient with gonorrhea may be treated with penicillin and probenecid (Benemid). Probenecid delays penicillin excretion, keeping this antibiotic in the body longer. **(M-S)**

▶ Pain that incapacitates a patient and can't be relieved by drugs is called *intractable pain*. **(IND)**

▶ In an emergency, consent for treatment can be obtained by fax, telephone, or other telegraphic transmission. **(FND)**

▶ In patients with glucose-6-phosphate dehydrogenase deficiency, the red blood cells can't metabolize adequate amounts of glucose; the condition results in hemolysis. **(M-S)**

▶ *Decibel* is the unit of measurement of sound. **(FND)**

▶ *On-call medication* refers to medication that should be ready for immediate administration when the call to administer it is received. **(M-S)**

▶ If gagging, nausea, or vomiting occurs when an airway is removed, the nurse should place the patient in a lateral position with the upper arm supported on a pillow. **(M-S)**

▶ *Emancipated minors* are individuals under the age of majority (usually age 18 or 21) who aren't under parental control, such as married minors, those who serve in the military, and college students who live away from home. **(PED)**

▶ Informed consent is required for any invasive procedure. **(FND)**

▶ A patient who can't write his or her name to give consent for treatment must have his or her X witnessed by two persons, such as a nurse, priest, or doctor. **(FND)**

▶ When a postoperative patient arrives in the recovery room, the nurse should position the patient on his side or with the head turned to the side and the chin extended. **(M-S)**

▶ In the immediate postoperative period, the nurse should report a respiratory rate greater than 30, temperature over 100° F (37.5° C) or below 97° F (36.5° C), or a significant drop in blood pressure or rise in pulse rate from the baseline. **(M-S)**

▶ Immunity to rubella can be measured by a hemagglutination inhibition test (rubella titer). This test identifies exposure to rubella infection and determines susceptibility to it in pregnant women (a woman has an immunity with a titer greater than 1:8). **(MAT)**

▶ In describing the degree of fetal descent during labor, floating occurs when the presenting part isn't engaged in the pelvic inlet but is freely movable (ballotable) above the pelvic inlet. **(MAT)**

▶ If the central nervous system is deprived of oxygen for more than 4 minutes, irreversible brain damage may occur. **(M-S)**

▶ In describing the degree of fetal descent, engagement occurs when the largest diameter of the presenting part has passed through the pelvic inlet. **(MAT)**

▶ The Z-track I.M. injection technique seals medication deep into the muscle, thereby minimizing skin irritation and staining. It requires a needle that is 1″ (2.5 cm) or longer. **(FND)**

▶ Fetal station (location of the presenting part) is described as –1, –2, –3, –4, or –5 to indicate the number of centimeters it is above the level of the ischial spines; station –5 is at the pelvic inlet. **(MAT)**

▶ Fetal station also is described as +1, +2, +3, +4, or +5 to indicate the number of centimeters it is below the level of the ischial spines; station 0 is at the level of the ischial spines. **(MAT)**

▶ During the first stage of labor, the side-lying position usually provides the greatest degree of comfort, although the patient may assume any position of comfort. **(MAT)**

▶ During delivery, if the umbilical cord can't be loosened and slipped from around the neonate's neck, it should be clamped with two clamps. Then the cord should be cut between the two clamps. **(MAT)**

▶ An Apgar score of 7 to 10 indicates no immediate distress, 4 to 6 indicates moderate distress, and 0 to 3 indicates severe distress. **(MAT)**

▶ Treatment for polycythemia vera includes administering oxygen, radioisotope therapy, or chemotherapy agents, such as chlorambucil and nitrogen mustard, to suppress bone marrow growth. **(M-S)**

▶ A patient with acute renal failure should receive a high-calorie diet that is low in protein and may be low in potassium and sodium. **(M-S)**

▶ Addison's disease results from adrenal gland hypofunction and is characterized by fatigue, anemia, weight loss, and bronze skin pigmentation. It usually is fatal without cortisol replacement therapy. **(M-S)**

▶ In the event of fire, the nurse should (1) remove the patient, (2) call the fire department, (3) attempt to contain the fire by closing the door, and (4) extinguish the fire, if it can be done safely. **(FND)**

▶ When caring for a depressed patient, the nurse's first priority is safety because of the increased risk of suicide. **(PSY)**

▶ Glaucoma is managed conservatively with beta-adrenergic blockers such as timolol (Timoptic), which decrease sympathetic impulses to the eye, and with miotic eyedrops such as pilocarpine (Isopto Carpine), which constrict the pupils. **(M-S)**

▶ Miotics effectively treat glaucoma by reducing intraocular pressure. They do this by constricting the pupil, contracting the ciliary muscles, opening the anterior chamber angle, and increasing the outflow of aqueous humor. **(M-S)**

▶ While a patient is receiving heparin, the nurse should monitor the partial thromboplastin time. **(M-S)**

▶ Urinary frequency, incontinence, or both can occur after catheter removal. Incontinence may be manifested as dribbling. **(M-S)**

▶ When teaching a patient about colostomy care, the nurse should instruct the patient to hang the irrigation reservoir 18″ to 22″ (45 to 55 cm) above the stoma, insert the catheter 2″ to 4″ (5 to 10 cm) into the stoma, irrigate the stoma with 17 to 34 oz (500 to 1,000 ml) of water at a temperature of 105° to 110° F (40° to 43° C) once a day, clean the area around the stoma with soap and water before applying a new bag, and use a protective skin covering, such as a Stomahesive wafer, karaya paste, or karaya ring, around the stoma. **(M-S)**

▶ The first sign of Hodgkin's disease is a painless, superficial lymphadenopathy, typically found under one arm or on one side of the neck in the cervical chain. **(M-S)**

▶ A registered nurse (RN) should assign a licensed vocational nurse (LVN) or licensed practical nurse (LPN) to perform bedside care, such as suctioning and medication administration. **(FND)**

▶ To differentiate "true cyanosis" from deposition of certain pigments, press over the discolored area; cyanotic skin blanches, pigmented skin doesn't.   **(M-S)**

▶ A patient with a gastric ulcer is most likely to report pain during or shortly after eating.   **(M-S)**

▶ A sign of increasing intracranial pressure is widening pulse pressure. For example, the blood pressure may rise from 120/80 to 160/60 mm Hg.   **(M-S)**

▶ In a burn victim, a primary goal of wound care is to prevent contamination by microorganisms.   **(M-S)**

▶ To prevent external rotation in a patient who has had hip nailing, the nurse places trochanter rolls from the knee to the ankle of the affected leg.   **(M-S)**

▶ Severe hip pain after the insertion of a hip prosthesis indicates dislodgment. If this occurs, the nurse should assess for shortening of the leg, external rotation, and absence of reflexes before calling the doctor.   **(M-S)**

▶ To elicit Moro's reflex, the nurse should hold the neonate in both hands and suddenly but gently drop the neonate's head backward. Normally, this causes the neonate to abduct and extend all extremities bilaterally and symmetrically, form a C shape with thumb and forefinger, and first adduct and then flex the extremities.   **(MAT)**

▶ *Echolalia* refers to the parrotlike repetition of another person's words or phrases.   **(PSY)**

▶ According to psychoanalytic theory, the ego is the part of the psyche that controls internal demands and interacts with the outside world at the conscious, preconscious, and unconscious levels.   **(PSY)**

▶ According to psychoanalytic theory, the superego is the part of the psyche that is composed of morals, values, and ethics. It is the aspect that continually evaluates thoughts and actions, rewarding the good and punishing the bad. (Think of the superego as the "supercop" of the unconscious.)   **(PSY)**

▶ According to psychoanalytic theory, the id is the part of the psyche that contains instinctual drives. (Remember *i* for instinctual and *d* for drive.) **(PSY)**

▶ According to Erikson, the child from birth to 12 months is in the trust-versus-mistrust stage of psychosocial development. **(PED)**

▶ Pregnancy-induced hypertension (preeclampsia) is defined as an increase in blood pressure of 30/15 mm Hg over baseline or a blood pressure of 140/95 mm Hg on two occasions at least 6 hours apart, edema, and albuminuria that occur after 20 weeks' gestation. **(MAT)**

▶ Positive signs of pregnancy include ultrasound evidence, fetal heart tones, and fetal movement felt by the examiner (not usually present until 4 months' gestation). **(MAT)**

▶ Goodell's sign is softening of the cervix. **(MAT)**

▶ Hegar's sign is softening of the lower uterine segment. **(MAT)**

▶ Quickening, a presumptive sign of pregnancy, occurs between 16 and 19 weeks' gestation. **(MAT)**

▶ Ovulation ceases during pregnancy. **(MAT)**

▶ Vaginal bleeding is the number one danger sign in pregnancy. **(MAT)**

▶ To estimate the date of confinement using Nägele's rule, the nurse counts backward 3 months from the first day of the last menstrual period and then adds 7 days to this date. **(MAT)**

▶ At 12 weeks' gestation, the fundus should be at the top of the symphysis pubis. **(MAT)**

▶ Koplik's spots are small, irregular red spots with minute bluish white centers that appear on the buccal mucosa of patients with measles (rubeola). **(PED)**

▶ Up to 75% of renal function must be lost before blood urea nitrogen and serum creatinine levels rise above normal. **(M-S)**

▶ When compensatory efforts are present in acid-base balance, the $Paco_2$ and the HCO_3^- will always point in the same direction:
pH↓ $Paco_2$↑ HCO_3^-↑ = respiratory acidosis compensated
pH↑ $Paco_2$↓ HCO_3^-↓ = respiratory alkalosis compensated
pH↓ $Paco_2$↓ HCO_3^-↓ = metabolic acidosis compensated
pH↑ $Paco_2$↑ HCO_3^+↑ = metabolic alkalosis compensated. **(M-S)**

▶ *Polyuria* refers to a urine output of 2,500 ml or more within 24 hours. **(M-S)**

▶ The therapeutic purpose of a mist tent is to increase hydration of secretions. **(FND)**

▶ The presenting sign of pleuritis is chest pain that is usually unilateral and related to respiratory movement. **(M-S)**

▶ If a patient can't void, the first nursing action should be bladder palpation to assess for bladder distention. **(FND)**

▶ If a patient has a gastric drainage tube in place, the nurse should expect the doctor to order potassium chloride. **(M-S)**

▶ Cow's milk shouldn't be given to infants under age 1 year because of its low linoleic acid content and its protein, which is difficult for infants to digest. **(MAT)**

▶ An increased pulse rate is one of the first indications of respiratory difficulty. It occurs because the heart attempts to compensate for a decreased oxygen supply to the tissues by pumping more blood. **(M-S)**

▶ If jaundice is suspected in a neonate, the nurse should examine the infant under natural light from a window. If natural light is unavailable, the nurse should examine the infant under a white light. **(MAT)**

▶ *Denial* refers to the defense mechanism used by a patient who denies the reality of an event. **(PSY)**

▶ The three phases of a uterine contraction are increment, acme, and decrement. **(MAT)**

▶ The patient who uses a cane should carry it on the unaffected side and advance it at the same time as the affected extremity. **(FND)**

▶ The patient with leg injury should advance the unaffected side first when climbing stairs and advance the affected leg first when descending stairs. **(M-S)**

▶ To fit a supine patient for crutches, the nurse should measure from the axilla to the sole and add 2″ (5 cm) to that measurement. **(FND)**

▶ A labor contraction's intensity can be assessed by the indentability of the uterine wall at the contraction's peak. Intensity is graded as mild (uterine muscle is somewhat tense), moderate (uterine muscle is moderately tense), or strong (uterine muscle is boardlike). **(MAT)**

▶ *Chloasma*, the mask of pregnancy, refers to skin pigmentation of a circumscribed area (usually over the bridge of the nose and cheeks) that is seen in some pregnancies. **(MAT)**

▶ The gynecoid pelvis is most ideal for delivery. Other types of pelves include platypelloid (flat), anthropoid (apelike), and android (malelike). **(MAT)**

▶ Pregnant women should be advised that there is no safe level of alcohol intake. **(MAT)**

▶ In an adult, a hemoglobin level below 11 mg/dl suggests that the patient has iron deficiency anemia and needs further evaluation. **(M-S)**

▶ The normal partial pressure of oxygen (PaO_2) in arterial blood is 95 mm Hg (plus or minus 5 mm Hg). **(M-S)**

▶ Vitamin C deficiency is characterized by brittle bones, pinpoint peripheral hemorrhages, and friable gums with loosened teeth. **(M-S)**

▶ Clinical manifestations of pulmonary embolism are extremely variable; however, increased respiratory rate, tachycardia, and hemoptysis are common. **(M-S)**

▶ In a psychiatric setting, seclusion is used to reduce overwhelming environmental stimulation, protect the patient from self-injury or injury to others, and prevent damage to hospital property. Used for patients who don't respond to less restrictive interventions, seclusion controls external behavior until the patient can assume self-control and supports the patient in re-gaining self-control.   **(PSY)**

▶ In a patient who takes a monoamine oxidase inhibitor, severe hypertension may occur if the patient eats tyramine-rich food, such as aged cheese, chicken liver, avocados, bananas, meat tenderizer, salami, bologna, Chianti wine, and beer.   **(PSY)**

▶ A patient who takes a monoamine oxidase inhibitor should be weighed biweekly and monitored for suicidal tendencies. If palpitations, headaches, or severe orthostatic hypotension oc-curs, the nurse should withhold the medication and notify the doctor.   **(PSY)**

▶ Normally, intraocular pressure ranges from 12 to 20 mm Hg. It can be measured with a Schiøtz tonometer.   **(M-S)**

▶ A uterine contraction's frequency is measured in minutes and represents the time from the beginning of one contraction to the beginning of the next.   **(MAT)**

▶ In early hemorrhagic shock, the patient's blood pressure may be normal, but the respiratory and pulse rates are rapid. The patient may complain of thirst, have clammy skin, and devel-op piloerection (goose bumps).   **(M-S)**

▶ Assessment begins with the nurse's first encounter with the pa-tient and continues throughout the patient's stay. The nurse obtains assessment data through the health history, physical examination, and review of diagnostic studies.   **(FND)**

▶ Cool, moist, pale skin, as occurs in shock, results from diver-sion of blood from the skin to the major organs.   **(M-S)**

▶ To assess capillary refill, the nurse applies pressure over the nail bed until blanching occurs, quickly releases the pressure, and notes the rate at which blanching fades. Capillary refill as-sesses perfusion, which decreases in shock, thereby lengthen-ing the refill time; a normal finding is less than 3 seconds.
                                                          (M-S)

▶ Except for patients with renal failure, low urine output signi-fies dehydration and the potential for shock.   **(M-S)**

▶ The appropriate needle size for an insulin injection is 25G and ⅝″ (1.5 cm) long.   **(FND)**

▶ *Residual urine* refers to urine that remains in the bladder after voiding. The amount of residual urine normally ranges from 50 to 100 ml.   **(FND)**

▶ The most common fracture in elderly patients is hip fracture. Osteoporosis weakens the bones, predisposing these patients to fracture, which usually results from a fall.   **(M-S)**

▶ The five stages of the nursing process are assessment, nursing diagnosis, planning, implementation, and evaluation.   **(FND)**

▶ *Planning* refers to the stage of the nursing process in which the nurse assigns priorities to nursing diagnoses, defines short-term and long-term goals and expected outcomes, and establishes the nursing care plan.   **(FND)**

▶ *Implementation* refers to the stage of the nursing process in which the nurse puts the nursing care plan into action, delegates specific nursing interventions to members of the nursing team, and charts patient responses to nursing interventions.   **(FND)**

▶ *Evaluation* refers to the stage of the nursing process in which the nurse compares objective and subjective data with the outcome criteria and, if needed, modifies the nursing care plan, making the nursing process circular.   **(FND)**

▶ Before angiography, ask the patient if he is allergic to the dye, shellfish, or iodine and advise him to take nothing by mouth for 8 hours before the procedure.   **(M-S)**

▶ During myelography, approximately 10 to 15 ml of cerebrospinal fluid is removed for laboratory studies and an equal amount of contrast media is injected.   **(M-S)**

▶ Vitamin K is administered to a newborn to prevent hemorrhagic fever because a newborn's intestine is unable to synthesize vitamin K.   **(MAT)**

▶ After angiography, the puncture site is covered with a pressure dressing and the affected part is immobilized for 8 hours to decrease the risk of bleeding.   **(M-S)**

▶ If a water-based medium was used during myelography, maintain the patient on bed rest for 6 to 8 hours with the head of the bed elevated 30 to 45 degrees. If an oil-based medium was used, keep the patient flat in bed for 6 to 24 hours. **(M-S)**

▶ The level of amputation is determined by estimating the maximum viable tissue (tissue with adequate circulation) needed to develop a functional stump. **(M-S)**

▶ Before internal fetal monitoring can be done, a pregnant patient's cervix must be dilated at least 2 cm, her amniotic membranes must be ruptured, and the fetus's presenting part (scalp or buttocks) must be at station –1 or lower, so that a small electrode can be attached to it. **(MAT)**

▶ Fetal alcohol syndrome presents in the first 24 hours after birth and produces lethargy, seizures, poor sucking reflex, abdominal distention, and respiratory difficulty. **(MAT)**

▶ *Variability* refers to any change in the fetal heart rate (FHR) from its normal rate of 120 to 160 beats/minute. An increased FHR is known as *acceleration*; a decreased FHR is known as *deceleration*. **(MAT)**

▶ Heparin sodium is in the dialysate used for renal dialysis. **(M-S)**

▶ Heroin withdrawal symptoms in a neonate may begin several hours to 4 days after birth. **(MAT)**

▶ Methadone withdrawal symptoms in a neonate may begin 7 days to several weeks after birth. **(MAT)**

▶ The cardinal signs of neonatal narcotic withdrawal include coarse flapping tremors, sleepiness, restlessness, prolonged and persistent high-pitched cry, and irritability. **(MAT)**

▶ The nurse should always count a neonate's respirations for 1 full minute. **(MAT)**

▶ Paroxysmal nocturnal dyspnea may indicate heart failure. **(M-S)**

▶ For a patient who takes a digitalis compound, such as digoxin or digitoxin, the diet should include high-potassium foods. **(M-S)**

▶ The nurse should limit tracheobronchial suctioning to 10 to 15 seconds and make only two passes. **(M-S)**

▶ Before performing tracheobronchial suctioning, the nurse should ventilate and oxygenate the patient five to six times with a resuscitation bag and 100% oxygen. This procedure is called *bagging*. **(M-S)**

▶ Signs and symptoms of pneumothorax include tachypnea, restlessness, hypotension, and tracheal deviation. **(M-S)**

▶ The first cardinal sign of toxic shock syndrome is rapid onset of a high fever. **(M-S)**

▶ A key sign of peptic ulcer is hematemesis, which can be bright red or dark red with the consistency of coffee grounds. **(M-S)**

▶ Signs and symptoms of a perforated peptic ulcer include sudden, severe upper abdominal pain; vomiting; and an extremely tender, rigid (boardlike) abdomen. **(M-S)**

▶ Constipation is a common adverse reaction to aluminum hydroxide. **(M-S)**

▶ For the first 24 hours after a myocardial infarction, a patient should use a bedside commode and then progress to walking to the toilet, bathing, and short walks. **(M-S)**

▶ Circumcision is postponed in neonates with hypospadias. **(MAT)**

▶ The post–myocardial infarction patient should avoid overexertion and add a new activity daily as tolerated without dyspnea. **(M-S)**

▶ In a patient who recently has had a myocardial infarction, frothy, blood-tinged sputum suggests pulmonary edema. **(M-S)**

▶ The primary purpose of drugs prescribed for a patient with acquired immunodeficiency syndrome is to prevent secondary infections. **(M-S)**

▶ Immune system suppression places a patient with acquired immunodeficiency syndrome at risk for developing opportunistic infections, such as cytomegalovirus, *Pneumocystis carinii* pneumonia, and thrush.   **(M-S)**

▶ A patient with acquired immunodeficiency syndrome may experience rapid weight loss, a sign of *wasting syndrome*.   **(M-S)**

▶ Between ages 10 and 12 months, a child begins to show emotions, such as affection, jealousy, and anger.   **(PED)**

▶ Chlorpromazine hydrochloride (Thorazine) is used to treat an infant who is addicted to narcotics.   **(MAT)**

▶ The nurse should use elbow restraints for protection on an infant with eczema or a scalp vein infusion or one who is recovering from cleft lip repair or eye surgery.   **(PED)**

▶ The nurse should provide a dark, quiet environment for an infant who is experiencing narcotic withdrawal.   **(MAT)**

▶ A good technique for assessing jaundice in a neonate is to blanch the tip of the nose or gum line by applying slight pressure under natural light and watching for yellow discoloration after removing pressure.   **(MAT)**

▶ The normal fasting blood glucose level in children is 60 to 100 mg/dl of blood.   **(PED)**

▶ If the body doesn't use glucose for energy, it metabolizes fat for energy, which results in ketone production.   **(M-S)**

▶ Separation from the mother evokes the most intense response in infants from age 6 to 12 months.   **(PED)**

▶ Because steroids mask symptoms of infection, they should be administered with extreme caution to children.   **(PED)**

▶ Steroids should be administered with food to a child.   **(PED)**

▶ Approximately 20% of patients with Guillain-Barré syndrome will have residual deficits such as mild motor weakness or diminished lower extremity reflexes.   **(M-S)**

▶ Signs and symptoms of leukemia in children include fatigue, anorexia, low-grade fever, and decreased white blood cell, red blood cell, and platelet counts. **(PED)**

▶ In children with leukemia, the most common causes of death include hemorrhage and infection. **(PED)**

▶ Anemia is the first sign of lead poisoning in a child. **(PED)**

▶ A Bradford frame is often used to immobilize a child with a spica cast. **(PED)**

▶ Signs of respiratory distress in a premature infant include nostril flaring, substernal retractions, and inspiratory grunting. **(MAT)**

▶ Hypertension and hypokalemia are the most significant clinical manifestations of primary hyperaldosteronism. **(M-S)**

▶ Having and frequently speaking to an imaginary friend are normal behaviors in a child age 3. **(PED)**

▶ An infant with normal motor development should be able to lift and control the head by 3 to 4 months. (Head lag is common in infants under 3 months.) **(PED)**

▶ Thrush is candidiasis *(Candida albicans)* of the oral mucous membranes. It is characterized by aphthae, or small ulcers, in the mouth. **(PED)**

▶ Common causes of child abuse are poor impulse control by parents and their lack of knowledge of growth and development. **(PSY)**

▶ Allopurinol (Zyloprim) is used in pediatric patients with leukemia to prevent uric acid accumulation. **(PED)**

▶ Before administering any as needed pain medication, the nurse should ask the patient to indicate the pain's location. **(FND)**

▶ At 6 months, an infant should begin to receive solid foods one at a time and 1 week apart. **(PED)**

▶ After percutaneous bladder aspiration, the patient's first void is usually pink; however, urine with frank blood should be reported to the doctor. **(M-S)**

▶ A urine culture that grows more than 100,000 colonies of bacteria per milliliter of urine demonstrates the existence of infection. **(M-S)**

▶ The most appropriate toy for a toddler age 18 months is one that helps develop motor coordination. **(PED)**

▶ When administering an injection to an infant, the nurse should ask another nurse to divert the child's attention and assist as needed. **(PED)**

▶ Premature infants develop respiratory distress syndrome (hyaline membrane disease) because their pulmonary alveoli lack surfactant. **(MAT)**

▶ Any time an infant is being put down to sleep, the mother should position the infant on the back (remember "back to sleep"). **(MAT)**

▶ A patient undergoing dialysis should take a vitamin supplement and eat foods that are high in calories but low in protein, sodium, and potassium. **(M-S)**

▶ The nurse should communicate at eye level with a child. **(PED)**

▶ An infant with phenylketonuria should have a low-phenylalanine formula and should have plasma phenylalanine levels monitored frequently. **(PED)**

▶ When caring for an infant who has had six to eight episodes of diarrhea a day for 4 days, the nurse should assess for electrolyte imbalance. **(PED)**

▶ The nurse may offer finger foods to a child age 3 who has a poor appetite. **(PED)**

▶ When in a mist tent (Croupette), a child may require soft restraints. **(PED)**

▶ In a patient with chronic obstructive pulmonary disease, the most effective ways to reduce thick secretions are to increase fluid intake to 2,500 ml/day and to encourage ambulation. **(M-S)**

▶ The nurse shouldn't administer medication to a child at bedtime unless specifically prescribed because it may stimulate the child. **(PED)**

▶ Medulloblastoma, the most common brain tumor in children, characteristically is found in the cerebellum. **(PED)**

▶ The nurse should teach a patient with emphysema how to perform pursed-lip breathing because it slows expiration, prevents alveolar collapse, and helps control the respiratory rate. **(M-S)**

▶ A patient with chronic obstructive pulmonary disease may develop clubbing of the digits and a barrel chest. **(M-S)**

▶ A cerebrovascular accident, a brain attack or stroke, disrupts the brain's blood supply and may be caused by hypertension. **(M-S)**

▶ Desired outcomes for a patient undergoing dialysis are normal weight, normal serum albumin levels (3.5 to 5.5 g/dl), and adequate protein intake (1.2 to 1.5 g/kg of body weight per day). **(M-S)**

▶ Intermittent peritoneal dialysis involves dialyzing for 40 hours/week in three to seven runs. **(M-S)**

▶ The best way to administer oxygen to a patient with chronic obstructive pulmonary disease is by nasal cannula; the normal flow rate is 2 to 3 L/minute. **(M-S)**

▶ Isoetharine hydrochloride (Bronkosol) can be administered by a handheld nebulizer or intermittent positive-pressure breathing. **(M-S)**

▶ *Brain death* refers to the irreversible cessation of brain function. **(M-S)**

▶ Continuous ambulatory peritoneal dialysis requires four exchanges a day, 7 days a week for a total of 168 hours a week. **(M-S)**

▶ The classic adverse reactions to antihistamines are dry mouth, drowsiness, and blurred vision. **(M-S)**

▶ A patient who has received a general anesthetic can't take anything by mouth until active bowel sounds are heard in all abdominal quadrants because of the risk of paralytic ileus. **(M-S)**

▶ Jehovah's Witnesses believe that they shouldn't receive blood components donated by other people. **(FND)**

▶ Alpha-fetoprotein is a tumor marker that is elevated in patients with testicular germ cell cancer. **(M-S)**

▶ Clinical manifestations of orchitis caused by bacteria or mumps are high temperature, chills, and sudden pain in the involved testis. **(M-S)**

▶ Prostate-specific antigen is elevated in benign prostatic hyperplasia and prostate cancer. **(M-S)**

▶ Prostatic acid phosphatase is elevated in advanced stages of prostate cancer. **(M-S)**

▶ Phenylephrine hydrochloride (Neo-Synephrine), a mydriatic, is instilled in a patient's eye to dilate the eye. **(M-S)**

▶ To test visual acuity, the nurse should ask the patient to cover each eye separately and read the eye chart with glasses and without, as appropriate. **(FND)**

▶ To promote fluid drainage and relieve edema in a patient with epididymitis, the nurse should elevate the scrotum on a scrotal bridge. **(M-S)**

▶ Fluorescein staining is commonly used to assess a corneal abrasion because it outlines superficial epithelial defects. **(M-S)**

▶ Presbyopia is a loss of near vision due to loss of elasticity of the crystalline lens. **(M-S)**

▶ When providing oral care for an unconscious patient, the nurse should position the patient on the side to minimize the risk of aspiration. **(FND)**

▶ During assessment of distance vision, the patient should stand 20′ (6.1 m) from the chart. **(FND)**

▶ Transient ischemic attacks are considered precursors to cerebrovascular accidents. **(M-S)**

▶ A sign of acute appendicitis, McBurney's sign is tenderness at McBurney's point (about 2″ [5 cm] from the right anterior superior iliac spine on a line between the spine and the umbilicus). **(M-S)**

▶ When caring for a patient with Guillain-Barré syndrome, the nurse should focus on respiratory interventions as the disease process advances. **(M-S)**

▶ The diagnosis of Alzheimer's disease is based on clinical findings of two or more cognitive deficits, progressive worsening of memory, and the results of a neuropsychological test. **(PSY)**

▶ Signs and symptoms of colon cancer include rectal bleeding, change in bowel habits, intestinal obstruction, abdominal pain, weight loss, anorexia, nausea, and vomiting. **(M-S)**

▶ Memory disturbance is a classic sign of Alzheimer's disease. **(PSY)**

▶ To help calm a child who is frightened of a mist tent, the nurse may suggest that a parent lie with the child in the tent. **(PED)**

▶ Symptoms of prostatitis include frequent urination and dysuria. **(M-S)**

▶ The male sperm contributes an X or a Y chromosome; the female ovum contributes an X chromosome. **(MAT)**

▶ Fertilization produces a total of 46 chromosomes, including an XY combination (male) or an XX combination (female). **(MAT)**

▶ A *chancre* is a painless, ulcerative lesion that develops during the primary stage of syphilis. **(M-S)**

▶ During the tertiary stage of syphilis, spirochetes invade the internal organs and cause permanent damage. **(M-S)**

▶ The ideal room temperature for a geriatric patient or one who is extremely ill ranges from 66° to 76° F (18.8° to 24.4° C). **(FND)**

▶ Normal room humidity ranges from 30% to 60%. **(FND)**

▶ Hand washing is the single best method of limiting the spread of microorganisms. Hands should be washed for 10 seconds after routine contact with a patient and after gloves are removed. **(FND)**

▶ The percentage of water in a newborn's body is about 78% to 80%. **(MAT)**

▶ In total parenteral nutrition, weight gain is the most reliable indicator of a positive response to therapy. **(M-S)**

▶ The nurse may administer an I.V. fat emulsion through a central or peripheral catheter but shouldn't use an in-line filter because the fat particles are too large to pass through the pores. **(M-S)**

▶ To catheterize a female patient, the nurse should place her in the dorsal recumbent position. **(FND)**

▶ A positive Homans' sign may indicate thrombophlebitis. **(FND)**

▶ Electrolytes in a solution are measured in milliequivalents per liter (mEq/L). A milliequivalent equals the number of milligrams per 100 milliliters of a solution. **(FND)**

▶ If a patient with a prostatectomy is using a Cunningham clamp, instruct him to wash and dry the penis before applying the clamp. He should apply the clamp horizontally and remove it at least every 4 hours to empty the bladder to prevent infection. **(M-S)**

▶ *Thought blocking* refers to loss of the train of thought because of a defect in mental processing. **(PSY)**

▶ A Bradford frame is used for a child who must be immobilized for a long period, such as one with extensive burns or meningocele. **(PED)**

▶ Metabolism takes place in two phases: anabolism (the constructive phase) and catabolism (the destructive phase). **(FND)**

▶ If a woman experiences signs of urinary tract infection during menopause, she should be instructed to drink six to eight glasses of water per day, urinate before and after intercourse, and perform Kegel exercises. **(M-S)**

▶ If a menopausal patient experiences a "hot flash," she should be instructed to seek a cool, breezy location and sip a cool drink. **(M-S)**

▶ The basal metabolic rate represents the amount of energy needed to maintain essential body functions. It is measured when the patient is awake and resting, hasn't eaten for 14 to 18 hours, and is in a comfortable, warm environment. **(FND)**

▶ The basal metabolic rate is expressed in calories consumed per hour per kilogram of body weight. **(FND)**

▶ Cheilosis produces fissures at the angles of the mouth and indicates a vitamin B_2, riboflavin, or iron deficiency. **(M-S)**

▶ Tetany may result from hypocalcemia secondary to hypoparathyroidism. **(M-S)**

▶ Dietary fiber (roughage), which is derived from cellulose, supplies bulk, maintains adequate intestinal motility, and helps establish regular bowel habits. **(FND)**

▶ Alcohol is metabolized primarily in the liver. Smaller amounts are metabolized by the kidneys and lungs. **(FND)**

▶ Inform the patient who has cervical cancer that she may experience vaginal bleeding for 1 to 3 months after intracavitary radiation. **(M-S)**

▶ Commonly caused by cirrhosis, *ascites* is the accumulation of fluid, which contains large amounts of protein and electrolytes, in the abdominal cavity. **(M-S)**

▶ Normal pulmonary artery pressure is 10 to 25 mm Hg and normal pulmonary wedge pressure is 5 to 12 mm Hg. **(M-S)**

▶ After cardiac catheterization, the site is monitored for bleeding and hematoma formation, pulses distal to the site are palpated every 15 minutes for 1 hour, and the patient is maintained on bed rest with the extremity extended for 8 hours. **(M-S)**

▶ Hemophilia is a bleeding disorder that is transmitted genetically in a sex-linked (X chromosome) recessive pattern. Although women may carry the defective gene, usually only men develop the disorder. **(M-S)**

▶ Von Willebrand's disease is an autosomal dominant bleeding disorder that results from platelet dysfunction and factor VIII deficiency. **(M-S)**

▶ Sickle cell anemia, a congenital hemolytic anemia, is caused by defective hemoglobin S molecules and primarily affects black patients. **(M-S)**

▶ Sickle cell anemia results from homozygous inheritance; sickle cell trait results from heterozygous inheritance. **(M-S)**

▶ A characteristic sign of Hodgkin's disease, Pel-Ebstein fever recurs every few days or weeks and alternates with afebrile periods. **(M-S)**

▶ *Petechiae* refers to tiny, round, purplish red spots that appear on the skin and mucous membranes as a result of intradermal or submucosal hemorrhage. **(FND)**

▶ *Purpura* refers to a purple skin discoloration caused by blood extravasation. **(FND)**

▶ Glucose-6-phosphate dehydrogenase (G6PD) deficiency is an inherited metabolic disorder characterized by red blood cells that are deficient in G6PD, a critical enzyme in aerobic glycolysis. **(M-S)**

▶ Preferred sites for bone marrow aspiration are the posterior superior iliac crest, anterior iliac crest, and sternum. **(M-S)**

▶ During bone marrow harvesting, the donor receives general anesthesia and 400 to 800 ml of marrow are aspirated. **(M-S)**

▶ A butterfly rash across the bridge of the nose is a characteristic sign of systemic lupus erythematosus. **(M-S)**

▶ Rheumatoid arthritis is a chronic, destructive collagen disease characterized by symmetric inflammation of the synovium, which leads to joint swelling. **(M-S)**

▶ A *compulsion* is an irresistible urge to perform an irrational act, such as walking in a clockwise circle before leaving a room or repeatedly washing hands. **(PSY)**

▶ A patient with a chosen method and a plan to commit suicide in the next 48 to 72 hours is at high risk for suicide. **(PSY)**

▶ Screening for human immunodeficiency virus antibodies begins with the enzyme-linked immunosorbent assay and is confirmed by the Western blot test. **(M-S)**

▶ The therapeutic serum level for lithium is 0.5 to 1.5 mEq/L. **(PSY)**

▶ Desensitization therapy, which gradually exposes a patient to an anxiety-producing stimulus, is used to treat phobic disorders. **(PSY)**

▶ *Dysfunctional grieving* refers to the absence of grief or grief that is prolonged beyond the usual time. **(PSY)**

▶ To perform nasotracheal suctioning in an infant, the nurse should position the infant with the neck slightly hyperextended in a "sniffing" position with the chin up and the head tilted back slightly. **(MAT)**

▶ The nurse should suction an infant quickly and gently to avoid hypoxia and apnea. (A longer period of suctioning may be used if the nurse administers oxygen by handheld resuscitation bag between suctioning periods.) **(PED)**

▶ Organogenesis occurs during the first trimester of pregnancy; specifically, days 14 to 56 of gestation. **(MAT)**

▶ After birth, the neonate's umbilical cord is tied 1″ (2.5 cm) from the abdominal wall with a cotton cord, plastic clamp, or rubber band. **(MAT)**

▶ The term *gravida* refers to the number of pregnancies regardless of their outcomes. **(MAT)**

▶ The term *para* refers to the number pregnancies that reached viability regardless of whether the fetus is delivered alive or stillborn. (A fetus is considered viable at 20 weeks' gestation.) **(MAT)**

▶ An *ectopic pregnancy* is one that implants abnormally, outside the uterus. **(MAT)**

▶ The first stage of labor begins with the onset of labor and ends with full cervical dilation at 10 cm. **(MAT)**

▶ The second stage of labor begins with full cervical dilation and ends with the neonate's birth. **(MAT)**

▶ The third stage of labor begins after the neonate's birth and ends with expulsion of the placenta. **(MAT)**

▶ In a full-term infant, skin creases appear over two-thirds of the newborn's feet. Heel creases of less than two-thirds are seen in preterm infants. **(MAT)**

▶ The fourth stage of labor (postpartal stabilization) lasts for up to 4 hours after delivery of the placenta (the time required to stabilize the mother's physical and emotional state after the stress of childbirth). **(MAT)**

▶ At 20 weeks' gestation, the fundus should be at the height of the umbilicus. **(MAT)**

▶ At 36 weeks' gestation, the fundus should be at the lower border of the rib cage. **(MAT)**

▶ A premature infant is one born before the end of the 37th week of gestation. **(MAT)**

▶ The creatine kinase MB-isoenzyme level elevates in 4 to 8 hours after a myocardial infarction, peaks at 12 to 24 hours, and returns to normal in 3 days. **(M-S)**

▶ During phase I of the nurse-patient relationship (beginning or orientation phase), an initial history is obtained and a mutual contract is agreed on. **(PSY)**

▶ During phase II of the nurse-patient relationship (middle or working phase), the patient discusses problems, behavioral changes occur, and self-defeating behavior is resolved or reduced. **(PSY)**

▶ During phase III of the nurse-patient relationship (termination or resolution phase), the nurse terminates the therapeutic relationship and gives the patient positive feedback on accomplishments. **(PSY)**

▶ Pregnancy-induced hypertension is a leading cause of maternal death in the United States. **(MAT)**

▶ A *habitual aborter* is a woman who has had three or more consecutive spontaneous abortions. **(MAT)**

▶ Threatened abortion occurs when bleeding is present without cervical dilation. **(MAT)**

▶ A complete abortion occurs when all products of conception have been expelled. **(MAT)**

▶ *Hydramnios* (polyhydramnios) refers to excessive amniotic fluid (more than 2,000 ml in the third trimester). **(MAT)**

▶ Excessive vitamin K intake may significantly antagonize the anticoagulant effects of warfarin (Coumadin). The patient should be cautioned against eating an excessive amount of leafy green vegetables. **(M-S)**

▶ According to the standard precautions recommended by the Centers for Disease Control and Prevention, the nurse shouldn't recap needles after use because most needle sticks result from missed needle recapping. **(FND)**

▶ According to Freud, a person between ages 12 and 20 is in the genital stage, during which he or she learns independence, has increased interest in members of the opposite sex, and establishes an identity. **(PSY)**

▶ According to Erikson, the identity-versus-role confusion stage occurs between ages 12 and 20. **(PSY)**

▶ *Tolerance* refers to the need for increasing amounts of a substance to achieve an effect that formerly was achieved with lesser amounts. **(PSY)**

▶ The antidote for heparin overdose is protamine sulfate. **(M-S)**

▶ A lymph node biopsy that shows Reed-Sternberg cells provides a definitive diagnosis of Hodgkin's disease. **(M-S)**

▶ The nurse should remove a child's mitts twice each shift to let the child exercise the fingers. **(PED)**

▶ Stress, dehydration, and fatigue may reduce a breast-feeding mother's milk supply. **(MAT)**

▶ *Bell's palsy* refers to unilateral facial weakness or paralysis caused by a disturbance of the seventh cranial (facial) nerve. **(M-S)**

▶ During the transition phase of the first stage of labor, the cervix is dilated 8 to 10 cm and contractions usually occur 2 to 3 minutes apart and last for 60 seconds. **(MAT)**

▶ A nonstress test is considered nonreactive (positive) if fewer than two fetal heart rate accelerations of at least 15 beats/minute occur in 20 minutes. **(MAT)**

▶ A nonstress test is considered reactive (negative) if two or more fetal heart rate accelerations of 15 beats/minute above baseline occur in 20 minutes. **(MAT)**

▶ A nonstress test usually is used to assess fetal well-being in a pregnant patient with a prolonged pregnancy (42 weeks or more), diabetes, a history of poor pregnancy outcomes, or pregnancy-induced hypertension. **(MAT)**

▶ The nurse administers a drug by I.V. push by delivering the dose directly into a vein, I.V. tubing, or catheter with a needle and syringe. **(FND)**

▶ When feeding an infant that has a tracheostomy tube, the nurse should cover the tracheostomy tube opening (stoma) with moistened gauze. (A bib may be used for a child over age 1.) **(PED)**

▶ When changing the ties on a tracheostomy tube, the nurse should leave the old ties in place until the new ones are applied. **(FND)**

▶ A nurse should have assistance when changing the ties on a tracheostomy tube. **(FND)**

▶ The nurse shouldn't lift an infant by the legs to change a diaper. She should roll the infant to the side, put the diaper in place, and then roll the infant back onto the diaper. **(PED)**

▶ A spica cast dries completely, from the outside to the inside, in 24 to 48 hours. **(PED)**

▶ During an initial tuberculin skin test, lack of a wheal after injection of tuberculin purified protein derivative indicates that the test dose was injected too deeply and that the nurse should inject another dose at least 2″ (5 cm) from the initial site. **(M-S)**

▶ A tuberculin skin test should be read 48 to 72 hours after administration. **(M-S)**

▶ In reading a tuberculin skin test, erythema without induration isn't generally significant. **(M-S)**

▶ Death from botulism usually results from delayed diagnosis and respiratory complications. **(M-S)**

▶ In a patient with rabies, saliva contains the rabies virus and constitutes a hazard for nurses who provide care. **(M-S)**

▶ A pregnant woman should drink at least eight 8-oz glasses (about 2,000 ml) of water daily. **(MAT)**

▶ A filter is always used for blood transfusions. **(FND)**

▶ The most common transfusion reaction is a febrile non-hemolytic reaction. **(M-S)**

▶ A four-point (quad) cane is indicated when a patient needs more stability than a regular cane can provide. **(FND)**

▶ The patient should carry a cane on the unaffected side to promote a reciprocal gait pattern and distribute weight away from the affected leg. **(FND)**

▶ A good way to begin a patient interview is to ask "What made you seek medical help?" **(FND)**

▶ The nurse should adhere to standard precautions for blood and body fluids when caring for all patients. **(FND)**

▶ Potassium (K^+) is the most abundant cation in intracellular fluid. **(FND)**

▶ Hypokalemia (abnormally low potassium concentration in the blood) may cause muscle weakness or paralysis, electrocardiographic abnormalities, and GI disturbances. **(M-S)**

▶ In the four-point gait (or alternating gait), the patient first moves the right crutch followed by the left foot and then the left crutch followed by the right foot. **(FND)**

▶ In the three-point gait, the patient moves two crutches and the affected leg simultaneously and then moves the unaffected leg. **(FND)**

▶ In the two-point gait, the patient moves the right leg and the left crutch simultaneously and then moves the left leg and the right crutch. **(FND)**

▶ Vitamin B complex, the water-soluble vitamins essential for metabolism, include thiamine (B_1), riboflavin (B_2), niacin (B_3), pyridoxine (B_6), and cyanocobalamin (B_{12}). **(FND)**

▶ When being weighed, an adult patient should be lightly dressed and shoeless. **(FND)**

▶ Beriberi disease, a serious vitamin B_1 (thiamine) deficiency, affects alcoholics with poor dietary habits and is epidemic in Asian countries where people subsist on unenriched rice. It is characterized by the phrase "I can't," indicating that the affected patient is too ill to do anything. **(M-S)**

▶ Before taking an adult's oral temperature, the nurse should ensure that the patient hasn't smoked or consumed hot or cold substances in the past 15 minutes. **(FND)**

▶ The nurse shouldn't take a rectal temperature on an adult patient if the patient has a cardiac disorder, anal lesions, or bleeding hemorrhoids or has recently undergone rectal surgery. **(FND)**

▶ Excessive sedation may cause respiratory depression. **(M-S)**

▶ In a patient with cardiac problems, rectal temperature measurement may stimulate a vagal response, leading to vasodilation and decreased cardiac output. **(FND)**

▶ When recording pulse amplitude and rhythm, the nurse should use these descriptive measures: +3 indicates a bounding pulse (readily palpable and forceful); +2, a normal pulse (easily palpable); +1, a thready or weak pulse (difficult to detect); and 0, an absent pulse (not detectable). **(FND)**

▶ A preoperative method of teaching a child about postoperative events is to describe them using a life-size doll that has an incision, a dressing, a cast, or an I.V. line, as appropriate. **(PED)**

▶ The intraoperative period begins when a patient is transferred to the operating room bed and ends when the patient is admitted to the postanesthesia recovery unit. **(FND)**

▶ On the morning of surgery, the nurse should ensure that the informed consent form has been signed; that the patient hasn't taken anything by mouth since midnight, has taken a shower with antimicrobial soap, has had mouth care (without swallowing the water), has removed common jewelry, and has received preoperative medication as prescribed; and that vital signs have been taken and recorded. Artificial limbs and other prostheses are usually removed. **(FND)**

▶ The primary postoperative concern is maintenance of a patent airway. **(M-S)**

▶ If cyanosis occurs circumorally, sublingually, or in the nail bed, the oxygen saturation level (SaO_2) is below 80%. **(M-S)**

▶ A rapid pulse rate in a postoperative patient may indicate pain, bleeding, dehydration, or shock. **(M-S)**

▶ Increased pulse rate and blood pressure may indicate that a patient is experiencing "silent pain" (pain that can't be expressed verbally, such as when a patient is recovering from anesthesia). **(M-S)**

▶ Lidocaine hydrochloride (Xylocaine) exerts antiarrhythmic action by suppressing automaticity in the Purkinje fibers and elevating electrical stimulation threshold in the ventricles. **(M-S)**

▶ Cullen's sign (a bluish discoloration around the umbilicus) is seen in patients with a perforated pancreas. **(M-S)**

▶ Comfort measures, such as positioning the patient, performing backrubs, and providing a restful environment, may decrease the patient's need for analgesics or may enhance their effectiveness. **(FND)**

▶ During the postoperative period, the patient should cough and deep breathe every 2 hours unless otherwise contraindicated (for example, craniotomy, cataract surgery, or throat surgery). **(M-S)**

▶ Before surgery, a patient's respiratory volume may be measured by incentive spirometry. This measurement becomes the patient's postoperative goal for respiratory volume. **(M-S)**

▶ The postoperative patient should use incentive spirometry 10 to 12 times per hour and take deep inhalations. **(M-S)**

▶ Before ambulating, a postoperative patient should dangle the legs over the side of the bed and perform deep-breathing exercises. **(M-S)**

▶ During the patient's first postoperative ambulation, the nurse should monitor closely and assist as needed while the patient walks a few feet from the bed to a steady chair. **(M-S)**

▶ Hypovolemia occurs when 15% to 25% of the body's total blood volume is lost. **(M-S)**

▶ Signs and symptoms of hypovolemia include rapid, weak pulse; low blood pressure; cool, clammy skin; shallow respirations; oliguria or anuria; and lethargy. **(M-S)**

▶ The clinical manifestation of acute pericarditis is sudden onset of severe and constant pain over the anterior chest that is aggravated by inspiration. **(M-S)**

▶ Signs and symptoms of septicemia include fever, chills, rash, abdominal distention, prostration, pain, headache, nausea, and diarrhea. **(M-S)**

▶ Rocky Mountain spotted fever can result from the bite of an infected wood tick or dog tick and produces a persistent high fever, nonpitting edema, and rash. **(M-S)**

▶ Advise patients who have undergone coronary artery bypass graft to sleep 6 to 10 hours per day, take their temperature twice per day, and avoid lifting more than 10 lb for at least 6 weeks. **(M-S)**

▶ Claudication pain (pain on ambulation) is caused by arterial insufficiency secondary to atheromatous plaque, which obstructs arterial blood flow to the extremities. **(M-S)**

▶ When both breasts are used for breast-feeding, the infant usually doesn't empty the second breast; therefore, the second breast should be used first at the next feeding. **(MAT)**

▶ Pacemakers can be powered by lithium batteries for up to 10 years. **(M-S)**

▶ The patient shouldn't void for 1 hour before percutaneous supra-pubic bladder aspiration to ensure that sufficient urine remains in the bladder to make the procedure successful. **(M-S)**

▶ Left-sided heart failure is manifested in pulmonary congestion, pink-tinged sputum, and dyspnea. (Think of L for left and lung.) **(M-S)**

▶ When applying a rubber band tourniquet on an infant's head in preparation for starting a scalp vein infusion, the nurse should place a second rubber band crosswise under the band to facilitate lifting and cutting the tourniquet when it is removed. **(PED)**

▶ A low-birth-weight infant is one who weighs 2,500 g (5 lb 8 oz) or less at birth. **(MAT)**

▶ A very-low-birth-weight infant is one who weighs 1,500 g (3 lb 5 oz) or less at birth. **(MAT)**

▶ When lifting an infant, the nurse should maintain two points of contact with the infant's body at all times. **(PED)**

▶ When teaching parents to provide umbilical cord care, the nurse should teach them to clean the umbilical area with alcohol on a cotton ball after every diaper change to prevent infection and promote drying. **(MAT)**

▶ Parents of young children should set their water heater thermostat no higher than 130° F (54° C). **(PED)**

▶ Suicide is the third leading cause of death among white teenagers. **(PSY)**

▶ Most teenagers who kill themselves had made a previous suicide attempt and had left telltale signs of their plans. **(PSY)**

▶ The nurse should teach a teenage girl that the most effective birth control method is abstinence and the second most effective method is oral contraceptive use. **(PED)**

▶ Teenage mothers are more likely to have low-birth-weight infants because they seek prenatal care late in their pregnancies (as a result of denial) and are more likely to have nutritional deficiencies. **(MAT)**

▶ Current recommended blood cholesterol level is less than 200 mg/dl. **(M-S)**

▶ When caring for a patient who is having a seizure, the nurse should follow these guidelines: (1) Avoid restraining the patient, but help a standing patient to a lying position. (2) Loosen restrictive clothing. (3) Place a pillow or other soft material under the patient's head. (4) Clear the area of hard objects. (5) Don't force anything into the patient's mouth, but maintain a patent airway. (6) Reassure and reorient the patient after the seizure subsides. **(M-S)**

▶ An adverse reaction to phenytoin (Dilantin) is gingival hyperplasia (also known as overgrowth of gum tissue). **(M-S)**

▶ A drug has three names: its generic name, which is used in official publications; its trade name or brand name (such as Tylenol), which is selected by the drug company; and its chemical name, which describes the drug's chemical composition. **(FND)**

▶ The patient should take a liquid iron preparation through a straw to avoid staining the teeth. **(FND)**

▶ The nurse should use the Z-track method to administer an I.M. injection of iron dextran (Imferon). **(FND)**

▶ An organism may enter the body through the nose, mouth, rectum, urinary or reproductive tract, or skin. **(FND)**

▶ With aging, most marrow in long bones becomes yellow but retains the capacity to convert back to red. **(M-S)**

▶ Clinical manifestations of lymphedema include fluid accumulation in the lower extremities. **(M-S)**

▶ *Afterload* is defined as ventricular wall tension during systolic ejection and can be increased in conditions that block aortic or pulmonary outflow, septal hypertrophy, and increased blood viscosity. **(M-S)**

▶ Red blood cells can be stored frozen for up to 2 years; however, they must be used within 24 hours of thawing. **(M-S)**

▶ Linea nigra, a dark line that extends from the umbilicus to the mons pubis, commonly appears during pregnancy and disappears after pregnancy. **(MAT)**

▶ Implantation in the uterus occurs 6 to 10 days after ovum fertilization. **(MAT)**

▶ In Erikson's stage of generativity versus despair, generativity (investment of self in the interest of the larger community) is expressed through procreation as well as through work, community service, and creative endeavors. **(PSY)**

▶ Most infants double their birth weight by age 5 to 6 months and triple it by age 1 year. **(PED)**

▶ For the first 24 hours after amputation, the nurse should elevate the patient's stump to prevent edema. **(M-S)**

▶ After hysterectomy, a woman should avoid sexual intercourse for 3 weeks if a vaginal approach was used and 6 weeks if the abdominal approach was used. **(M-S)**

▶ In descending order, the levels of consciousness are alertness, lethargy, stupor, light coma, and deep coma. **(FND)**

▶ Parkinson's disease characteristically produces progressive muscle rigidity, akinesia, and involuntary tremor. **(M-S)**

▶ Tonic-clonic seizures are characterized by a loss of consciousness and alternating periods of muscle contraction and relaxation. **(M-S)**

▶ Status epilepticus, a life-threatening emergency, is a series of rapidly repeating seizures without intervening periods of consciousness. **(M-S)**

▶ The ideal donor for a kidney transplantation is a twin. If a twin isn't available, a biological sibling is the next best choice. **(M-S)**

▶ Breast cancer is the leading cancer among women; however, lung cancer accounts for more deaths. **(M-S)**

▶ The stages of cervical cancer are stage 0, carcinoma in situ; stage I, cancer confined to the cervix; stage II, cancer extension beyond the cervix but not to the pelvic wall; stage III, cancer extension to the pelvic wall; and stage IV, cancer extension beyond the pelvis or within the bladder or rectum. **(M-S)**

▶ One method of estimating blood loss after a hysterectomy is by counting perineal pads. Saturating more than one pad an hour or eight in 24 hours is considered hemorrhaging. **(M-S)**

▶ Transurethral resection of the prostate is the most common procedure for treating benign prostatic hyperplasia. **(M-S)**

▶ In a chest drainage system, the water in the water-seal chamber normally rises when a patient breathes in and falls when he breathes out. **(M-S)**

▶ *Placenta previa* refers to the abnormally low implantation of the placenta so that it encroaches on or covers the cervical os. **(MAT)**

▶ Spinal fusion provides spinal stability through a bone graft, usually from the iliac crest, that fuses two or more vertebrae. **(M-S)**

▶ To turn a patient by logrolling, the nurse folds the patient's arms across the chest; extends the patient's legs and inserts a pillow between them, if indicated; places a draw sheet under the patient; and turns the patient by slowly and gently pulling on the draw sheet. **(FND)**

▶ In complete (total) placenta previa, the placenta completely covers the cervical os. **(MAT)**

▶ In partial (incomplete or marginal) placenta previa, the placenta covers only a portion of the cervical os. **(MAT)**

▶ A patient who receives any type of transplant must receive an immunosuppressant drug for life. **(M-S)**

▶ *Abruptio placentae* refers to the premature separation of a normally implanted placenta. It may be partial or complete and usually causes abdominal pain, vaginal bleeding, and a boardlike abdomen. **(MAT)**

▶ *Cutis marmorata* (mottling or purple skin discoloration) refers to a transient vasomotor response that occurs primarily in the arms and legs of infants exposed to cold. **(MAT)**

▶ The classic triad of symptoms of preeclampsia are hypertension, edema, and proteinuria. Additional symptoms in severe preeclampsia include hyperreflexia, cerebral and visual disturbances, and epigastric pain. **(MAT)**

▶ Incentive spirometry should be used 5 to 10 times an hour while awake. **(M-S)**

▶ In a male patient who has reached puberty, the major complication of mumps is sterility caused by orchitis. **(PED)**

▶ Pelvic inflammatory disease is a common complication of gonorrhea in women. **(M-S)**

▶ Hirschsprung's disease (congenital megacolon) is the congenital absence of parasympathetic ganglia in the distal portion of the colon and rectum, which results in a lack of peristalsis. **(PED)**

▶ Ortolani's sign (an audible click or palpable jerk with thigh abduction) confirms congenital hip dislocation in a neonate. **(MAT)**

▶ *Scoliosis* refers to a lateral S-shaped curvature of the spine. **(M-S)**

▶ According to Freud, conflicts that arise in the phallic stage (Oedipus or Electra complex) are resolved when the child identifies with the parent of the same sex. **(PED)**

▶ Signs and symptoms of the secondary stage of syphilis include a rash on the palms and soles, erosion of the oral mucosa, alopecia, and enlarged lymph nodes. **(M-S)**

▶ Alcoholics Anonymous recommends a 12-step program to achieve sobriety. **(PSY)**

▶ The nurse should monitor glucose and electrolyte levels in a patient receiving total parenteral nutrition. **(M-S)**

▶ Signs and symptoms of anorexia nervosa include amenorrhea, excessive weight loss, lanugo (fine body hair), abdominal distention, and electrolyte disturbances. **(PSY)**

▶ Unless contraindicated, on admission to the postanesthesia care unit, a patient should be turned on his side first and then his vital signs should be taken. **(M-S)**

▶ Edema is treated by limiting fluid intake and eliminating excess fluid. **(M-S)**

▶ Keep the patient who has had spinal anesthesia flat for 12 to 24 hours and monitor vital signs and neuromuscular function. **(M-S)**

▶ Serum lithium levels that exceed 2.0 mEq/L are considered toxic. **(PSY)**

▶ A patient with maple syrup urine disease should avoid food containing the amino acids leucine, isoleucine, and lysine. **(M-S)**

▶ A severe complication of a femur fracture is excessive blood loss, resulting in shock. **(M-S)**

▶ To prepare the patient for peritoneal dialysis, the nurse should ask the patient to void, measure the patient's vital signs, place the patient in a supine position and, using aseptic technique, insert a catheter through the abdominal wall into the peritoneal space. **(M-S)**

▶ If more than 3 L of dialysate solution return during peritoneal dialysis, the nurse should notify the doctor. **(M-S)**

▶ *Hemodialysis* is the removal of certain elements from the blood by passing heparinized blood through a semipermeable membrane to the dialysate bath, which contains all the important electrolytes in their ideal concentrations. **(M-S)**

▶ The first immunization for a newborn is the hepatitis B vaccine, which is given in the nursery shortly after birth. **(MAT)**

▶ Gangrene usually affects the digits first and begins with skin color changes that progress from gray-blue to dark brown or black. **(M-S)**

▶ Kidney function is assessed by evaluating blood urea nitrogen (normal range is 8 to 20 mg/dl) and serum creatinine (normal range is 0.6 to 1.3 mg/dl) levels. **(M-S)**

▶ The diaphragm of the stethoscope is used to hear high-pitched sounds such as breath sounds. **(FND)**

▶ A slight blood pressure difference (5 to 10 mm Hg) between right and left arms is normal. **(FND)**

▶ A weight-bearing transfer is appropriate only for a patient who has at least one leg that is strong enough to bear weight, such as a patient with hemiplegia or a single leg amputation. **(M-S)**

▶ The nurse should place the blood pressure cuff 1″ (2.5 cm) above the antecubital fossa. **(FND)**

▶ When instilling ophthalmic ointments, waste the first bead of ointment and then apply from the inner canthus to the outer canthus; twist the medication tube to detach the ointment. **(FND)**

▶ The nurse should use a leg cuff to measure blood pressure in an obese patient. **(FND)**

▶ If the blood pressure cuff is applied too loosely, the reading will be falsely elevated. **(FND)**

▶ *Ptosis* refers to eyelid drooping. **(FND)**

▶ Overflow incontinence (voiding of 30 to 60 ml of urine every 15 to 30 minutes) is a sign of bladder distention. **(M-S)**

▶ The first sign of a pressure ulcer is reddened skin that blanches when pressure is applied. **(M-S)**

▶ A tilt table is useful for a patient with a spinal cord injury, orthostatic hypotension, or brain damage because it can move the patient gradually from a horizontal to a vertical (upright) position. **(FND)**

▶ To perform venipuncture with the least injury to the vessel, the nurse should turn the bevel upward when the vessel's lumen is larger than the needle and turn it downward when the lumen is only slightly larger than the needle. **(FND)**

▶ To move the patient to the edge of the bed for transfer, follow these steps: (1) Move the patient's head and shoulders toward the edge of the bed. (2) Move the patient's feet and legs to the edge of the bed (crescent position). (3) Place both arms well under the patient's hips and straighten the back while moving the patient toward the edge of the bed. **(FND)**

► Late signs and symptoms of sickle cell anemia include tachycardia, cardiomegaly, systolic and diastolic murmurs, chronic fatigue, hepatomegaly, and splenomegaly. **(M-S)**

► Signs and symptoms of sickle cell anemia during early childhood include jaundice, pallor, joint swelling, bone pain, chest pain, ischemic leg ulcers, and an increased susceptibility to infection. **(PED)**

► When being measured for crutches, a patient should wear his or her shoes. **(FND)**

► If a patient misses a menstrual period while taking an oral contraceptive exactly as prescribed, she should continue taking the contraceptive. **(MAT)**

► If a patient misses two consecutive menstrual periods while taking an oral contraceptive, she should discontinue the contraceptive and have a pregnancy test. **(MAT)**

► If a patient taking an oral contraceptive misses a dose, she should take the pill as soon as she remembers or take two at the next scheduled interval and continue with the normal schedule. **(MAT)**

► If a patient taking an oral contraceptive misses two consecutive doses, she should double the dose for 2 days and then resume her normal schedule. She should also use an additional birth control method for 1 week. **(MAT)**

► A mechanical ventilator, which can maintain ventilation automatically for an extended period, is indicated when a patient can't maintain a safe Pao_2 or $Paco_2$ level. **(M-S)**

► Two types of mechanical ventilators exist: negative-pressure ventilators, which apply negative pressure around the chest wall, and positive-pressure ventilators, which deliver air under pressure to the patient. **(M-S)**

► Angina pectoris is characterized by substernal pain that lasts for 2 to 3 minutes. The pain, which is caused by myocardial ischemia, may radiate to the neck, shoulders, or jaw; is described as viselike or constricting; and may be accompanied by severe apprehension or a feeling of impending doom. **(M-S)**

▶ Anginal pain that persists for more than 20 minutes and isn't relieved by nitroglycerin indicates a developing myocardial infarction. **(M-S)**

▶ The goal of treatment for a patient with angina pectoris is to reduce the heart's workload, thereby reducing the myocardial oxygen demand and preventing myocardial infarction. **(M-S)**

▶ Nitroglycerin decreases the amount of blood returning to the heart by increasing the capacity of the venous bed. **(M-S)**

▶ The patient should take no more than three nitroglycerin tablets in a 15-minute period. **(M-S)**

▶ Hemodialysis usually is performed 24 hours before kidney transplantation. **(M-S)**

▶ Signs and symptoms of acute kidney transplant rejection are progressive enlargement and tenderness at the transplant site, increased blood pressure, decreased urine output, elevated serum creatinine level, and fever. **(M-S)**

▶ In an infant, one of the first signs of dehydration is sunken fontanels. **(PED)**

▶ After a radical mastectomy, the patient's arm should be elevated (hand above elbow) on a pillow to enhance circulation and prevent edema. **(M-S)**

▶ Postoperative mastectomy care includes teaching the patient arm exercises to facilitate lymph drainage and prevent muscle shortening and shoulder joint contracture (frozen shoulder). **(M-S)**

▶ *Eclampsia* is the occurrence of seizures not caused by a cerebral disorder in a patient with pregnancy-induced hypertension. **(MAT)**

▶ A patient who has had a radical mastectomy should help prevent infection by making sure that no blood pressure readings, injections, or venipunctures are performed on the affected arm. **(M-S)**

► In placenta previa, bleeding is painless and seldom fatal on the first occasion but becomes heavier with each subsequent episode. **(MAT)**

► For a mastectomy patient prone to lymphedema, the hand exercise program can begin shortly after surgery, if prescribed. It consists of having the patient open and close her hand tightly six to eight times hourly and perform such tasks as washing her face and combing her hair. **(M-S)**

► Treatment for abruptio placentae usually is immediate cesarean section. **(MAT)**

► The nurse should transport a hospitalized infant or child in a stroller, wheelchair, or bed, rather than hand-carry the infant or child. **(PED)**

► The nurse should attach a restraint to the part of the bed frame that moves with the head, not to the mattress or side rails. **(FND)**

► Drugs used to treat neonatal withdrawal symptoms include phenobarbital (Luminal), camphorated opium tincture (paregoric), and diazepam (Valium). **(MAT)**

► Signs and symptoms of theophylline toxicity include vomiting, restlessness, and an apical pulse rate over 200 beats/minute. **(M-S)**

► The mist in a mist tent should never become so dense that it obscures clear visualization of the patient's respiratory pattern. **(FND)**

► The nurse should teach the parent of a child with croup not to administer cough medication because it may worsen the child's respiratory distress by inhibiting the body's natural response to clear the throat by coughing. **(PED)**

► Infants with Down syndrome typically display marked hypotonia, floppiness, slanted eyes, excess skin on the back of the neck, flattened bridge of the nose, flat facial features, spadelike hands, short and broad feet, small male genitalia, absence of Moro's reflex, and a simian crease on the hands. **(MAT)**

▶ The nurse shouldn't induce vomiting in a person who has ingested poison and is having seizures or is semiconscious or comatose. **(M-S)**

▶ Public Law 94-247 (Child Abuse and Neglect Act of 1973) requires that suspected cases of child abuse be reported to child protection services. **(PSY)**

▶ The nurse should suspect sexual abuse in a young child who has blood in the stool or urine, penile or vaginal discharge, genital trauma that isn't readily explained, or a sexually transmitted disease. **(PSY)**

▶ Central venous pressure, the pressure in the right atrium and the great veins in the thorax, normally ranges from 2 to 8 mm Hg (or 5 to 12 cm of water) and serves as a guide for assessing right-sided cardiac function. **(M-S)**

▶ Central venous pressure monitoring is used to assess the need for fluid replacement in seriously ill patients, estimate blood volume deficits, and evaluate circulatory pressure in the right atrium. **(M-S)**

▶ To administer heparin subcutaneously, the nurse should follow these steps: (1) Clean, but don't rub, the site with alcohol. (2) Stretch the skin taut or pick up a well-defined skin fold. (3) Hold the shaft of the needle in a dart position. (4) Insert the needle into the skin at a right (90-degree) angle. (5) Firmly depress the plunger, but don't aspirate. (6) Leave the needle in place for 10 seconds. (7) Withdraw the needle gently at the same angle it was inserted. (8) Apply pressure to the injection site with an alcohol pad. **(FND)**

▶ To prevent deep vein thrombosis after surgery, the nurse should administer 5,000 units of heparin subcutaneously every 8 to 12 hours, as prescribed. **(M-S)**

▶ Oral anticoagulants, such as warfarin sodium (Coumadin) and dicumarol, disrupt natural blood clotting mechanisms, prevent thrombus formation, and limit the extension of a formed thrombus. **(M-S)**

▶ Anticoagulants can't dissolve a formed thrombus. **(M-S)**

▶ Anticoagulant therapy is contraindicated in a patient with liver or kidney disease or GI ulcers or a patient who isn't likely to return for follow-up visits. **(M-S)**

▶ The nurse can assess for thrombophlebitis by measuring the patient's affected and unaffected legs and comparing their sizes. The nurse should mark measurement locations with a pen so that the measurements can be taken at the same place each day. **(M-S)**

▶ Drainage of more than 3,000 ml of fluid daily from a nasogastric tube may suggest intestinal obstruction. Yellow drainage with a foul odor may indicate small-bowel obstruction. **(M-S)**

▶ For a sigmoidoscopy, the nurse should place the patient in a knee-chest or Sims' position, depending on the doctor's preference. **(FND)**

▶ Preparation for sigmoidoscopy includes administering an enema 1 hour before the examination, warming the scope in warm water or a sterilizer (if using a metal sigmoidoscope), and draping the patient so that the perineum is exposed. **(M-S)**

▶ Treatment for a patient with bleeding esophageal varices includes administering vasopressin (Pitressin), giving an ice water lavage, aspirating blood from the stomach, using esophageal balloon tamponade, providing parenteral nutrition, and administering blood transfusions, as needed. **(M-S)**

▶ A trauma victim shouldn't be moved until a patent airway has been established and the cervical spine has been immobilized. **(M-S)**

▶ After a mastectomy, lymphedema may cause a feeling of heaviness in the arm. **(M-S)**

▶ A school-age child faced with dying should be told the truth. The child should receive an explanation of the diagnosis and should be allowed to die in comfort surrounded by family. **(PED)**

▶ A preschool-age child with a fatal disease isn't likely to ask if he or she is going to die but may express anxiety about death through play therapy or other activities. Most developmental theorists recommend helping such a child by responding honestly to questions and providing reassurance that he or she won't be alone. **(PED)**

▶ It is appropriate for the parents and family to tell their dying child that they will miss him or her and that they are sad because they will be separated. **(PED)**

▶ An adolescent with a terminal illness should be told the truth about the prognosis, although resentment and denial ("Is it possible that I will live?") are common responses. **(PED)**

▶ A dying patient shouldn't be given an absolute time left to live but should receive a statement such as "Some people live 3 to 6 months, but others live longer." **(M-S)**

▶ After a child dies, the nurse should give family members time with the body, compliment them (as appropriate) on the excellent care they provided, and give them the name of a person to contact if they have questions. **(PED)**

▶ Amniocentesis (needle aspiration of amniotic fluid) usually is performed at 15 to 17 weeks' gestation to detect fetal abnormalities. **(MAT)**

▶ For a child over age 1 who has ingested a noncorrosive poison, treatment should include administration of 15 ml of syrup of ipecac mixed in warm water. If the first dose is ineffective, a second dose may be ordered by the doctor. Tincture of ipecac shouldn't be used because it is stronger than syrup of ipecac and is itself a poison. **(PED)**

▶ After eye surgery, a patient should avoid using makeup until otherwise instructed. **(M-S)**

▶ After a corneal transplant, the patient should wear an eye shield when engaging in activities such as playing with children or pets. **(M-S)**

▶ After a corneal transplant, the patient shouldn't lay on the operative site, bend at the waist, or have sexual intercourse for 1 week. The patient should always avoid getting soap suds in the eye. **(M-S)**

▶ An alcoholic uses alcohol as a way to cope with the stresses of life. **(PSY)**

▶ Theophylline, steroids, and terbutaline commonly are used to treat children with asthma. **(PED)**

▶ Treatment of a child with celiac disease includes following a lifelong gluten-free diet. (Gluten is found in wheat, oats, and barley.) **(PED)**

▶ The *ectoderm* is the outermost layer of the three primary germ layers of the embryo. **(MAT)**

▶ The human personality operates on three levels: conscious, preconscious, and unconscious. **(PSY)**

▶ Asking an open-ended question is one of the best ways to elicit or clarify information from a patient. **(PSY)**

▶ The failure rate of a contraceptive is determined by the experience of 100 women for 1 year and is expressed as pregnancies per 100 women years. **(MAT)**

▶ The narrowest diameter of the pelvic inlet is the anteroposterior (diagonal conjugate). **(MAT)**

▶ The *chorion* is the outermost extraembryonic membrane that gives rise to the placenta. **(MAT)**

▶ The corpus luteum secretes large quantities of progesterone. **(MAT)**

▶ From the 8th week of gestation through delivery, the developing cells are termed a *fetus*. **(MAT)**

▶ The diagnosis of autism is often made when a child is between ages 2 and 3. **(PSY)**

▶ In an incomplete abortion, the fetus is expelled but parts of the placenta and membrane remain in the uterus. **(MAT)**

▶ A neonate's head circumference is normally 2 to 3 cm greater than the chest circumference. **(MAT)**

▶ After administering magnesium sulfate to a pregnant patient for hypertension or preterm labor, the nurse should monitor her respiratory rate and deep tendon reflexes. **(MAT)**

▶ During the first hour after birth (the period of reactivity), the neonate is alert and awake. **(MAT)**

▶ When a pregnant patient has undiagnosed vaginal bleeding, vaginal examinations should be avoided until ultrasonography rules out placenta previa. **(MAT)**

▶ After a neonate is delivered, the first nursing action is to establish the neonate's airway. **(MAT)**

▶ Nursing interventions for a patient with placenta previa include positioning the patient on her left side for maximum fetal perfusion, monitoring fetal heart tones, and administering I.V. fluids and oxygen, as ordered. **(MAT)**

▶ When taking a child's temperature rectally, the nurse should insert the thermometer only ½" (1.3 cm). **(PED)**

▶ The specific gravity of a neonate's urine is 1.003 to 1.030. A lower specific gravity suggests overhydration; a higher one suggests dehydration. **(MAT)**

▶ During the oral stage of development (from age 1 to 18 months), the infant receives satisfaction, relieves tension, and derives pleasure from sucking and chewing. **(PED)**

▶ Defense mechanisms serve as protectors of the personality by reducing stress and anxiety. **(PSY)**

▶ A Milwaukee brace, which is used for patients with structural scoliosis, helps halt the progression of spinal curvature by providing longitudinal traction and lateral pressure. It should be worn 23 hours a day. **(M-S)**

▶ *Suppression* refers to the voluntary act of excluding anxiety- or stress-producing thoughts from the conscious. **(PSY)**

▶ Most infants are weighed and measured monthly for the first 6 months of life. **(PED)**

▶ The neonatal period extends from birth to day 28. It may also be called the first 4 weeks or first month of life. **(MAT)**

▶ The infancy period lasts from birth to age 1. **(PED)**

▶ The toddler stage encompasses ages 1 to 3. **(PED)**

▶ Children with chronic protein-calorie malnutrition are small for their age, physically inactive, mentally sluggish, and susceptible to infections.   **(PED)**

▶ Short-term measures for stomal retraction include stool softeners, irrigations, and stomal dilatation.   **(M-S)**

▶ A woman who is breast-feeding should rub a mild emollient cream or a few drops of breast milk (or colostrum) on the nipples after each feeding and let breasts air-dry to prevent them from cracking.   **(MAT)**

▶ Breast-feeding mothers should increase their fluid intake to 2.5 to 3 qt (2,500 to 3,000 ml) daily.   **(MAT)**

▶ Psychodrama is a therapeutic technique used with groups to help participants gain new perception and self-awareness by acting out their own or assigned problems.   **(PSY)**

▶ Maslow's hierarchy of needs must be met in the following order: physiologic (oxygen, food, water, sex, rest, and comfort), safety and security, love and belonging, self-esteem and recognition, and self-actualization.   **(FND)**

▶ A patient who is taking disulfiram (Antabuse) must avoid ingesting products that contain alcohol, such as cough syrup, fruitcake, and sauces and soups made with cooking wine.   **(PSY)**

▶ A patient who is admitted involuntarily to a psychiatric hospital loses the right to sign out against medical advice.   **(PSY)**

▶ "People who live in glass houses shouldn't throw stones" and "A rolling stone gathers no moss" are examples of proverbs used during a psychiatric interview to determine a patient's ability to think abstractly. (Schizophrenic patients think in concrete terms and might interpret the glass house proverb as "If you throw a stone in a glass house, the house will break.")   **(PSY)**

▶ Signs of lithium toxicity include diarrhea, tremors, nausea, muscle weakness, ataxia, and confusion.   **(PSY)**

▶ A labile affect is characterized by rapid shifts of emotions and mood.   **(PSY)**

▶ *Amnesia* refers to a loss of memory from an organic or inorganic cause. **(PSY)**

▶ A person with borderline personality disorder is demanding and judgmental in interpersonal relationships and will attempt to split staff by pointing to discrepancies in the treatment plan. **(PSY)**

▶ Disulfiram (Antabuse) shouldn't be taken concurrently with metronidazole (Flagyl) because they may interact, causing a psychotic reaction. **(PSY)**

▶ Congenital hip dysplasia is the most common disorder of the hip joint in a patient under age 3. **(PED)**

▶ A patient with a colostomy should be advised to eat a low-residue diet for 4 to 6 weeks, then to add one food at a time to evaluate its effect. **(M-S)**

▶ To relieve postoperative hiccups, the patient should rebreathe into a paper bag. **(M-S)**

▶ If a patient with an ileostomy has a blocked lumen from undigested, high-fiber food, place the patient in the knee-chest position and massage the area below the stoma. **(M-S)**

▶ After feeding an infant with a cleft lip or palate, the nurse should rinse the infant's mouth with sterile water. **(MAT)**

▶ An infant with a cleft palate is at increased risk of developing otitis media. **(PED)**

▶ When examining an infant's ear with an otoscope, the nurse should pull the earlobe down and back. **(PED)**

▶ The nurse should place oral medication to the side of the mouth in an infant who has had corrective surgery for a cleft lip or palate. **(PED)**

▶ The nurse should position a child with meningococcal meningitis on the side if opisthotonos (back arching) occurs. **(PED)**

▶ Between ages 2 and 3, a child engages in parallel play and begins to interact with others. **(PED)**

► For a child with ascites from a chronic liver disease, the nurse should use semi-Fowler's position to promote respiratory functioning. **(PED)**

► An autistic child is difficult to understand because of withdrawal, unresponsiveness, and severely impaired speech. **(PED)**

► In a toddler, the first signs of respiratory distress are increased respiratory and pulse rates. **(PED)**

► Toilet training usually is unsuccessful before ages 15 to 18 months because sphincter control develops at this age. **(PED)**

► The nurse instills erythromycin in the neonate's eyes primarily to prevent blindness caused by gonorrhea or chlamydia. **(MAT)**

► Because gonorrhea is asymptomatic and progresses without detection in most teenage girls, their fallopian tubes can be damaged. **(PED)**

► During the initial interview and treatment of a patient with syphilis, the patient's sexual contacts should be identified. **(M-S)**

► The nurse shouldn't administer morphine to a patient whose respiratory rate has fallen below 12 breaths/minute. **(M-S)**

► Oxygen should be administered with hydration in order to prevent drying of the mucous membranes. **(M-S)**

► Flavoxate hydrochloride (Urispas) is classified as a urinary tract spasmolytic. **(M-S)**

► Hypotension is a sign of cardiogenic shock in a patient with a myocardial infarction. **(M-S)**

► The predominant signs of mechanical ileus are cramping pain, vomiting, distention, and inability to pass stools or flatus. **(M-S)**

► For a patient with a myocardial infarction, the nurse should monitor fluid intake and output meticulously because too little intake causes dehydration and too much may cause pulmonary edema. **(M-S)**

► Nitroglycerin relaxes smooth muscle, causing vasodilation and relieving the chest pain associated with myocardial infarction and angina. **(M-S)**

▶ The diagnosis of an acute myocardial infarction is based on the patient's signs and symptoms, electrocardiogram tracings, and serum enzyme studies. **(M-S)**

▶ Arrhythmias are the predominant problem during the first 48 hours after a myocardial infarction. **(M-S)**

▶ Clinical manifestations of malabsorption include weight loss, muscle wasting, bloating, and steatorrhea. **(M-S)**

▶ When caring for a patient with a nasogastric tube, the nurse should apply a water-soluble lubricant to the nostril to prevent soreness. **(FND)**

▶ Asparaginase, an enzyme that inhibits deoxyribonucleic acid and protein synthesis, is used to treat acute lymphocytic leukemia. **(M-S)**

▶ To relieve a patient's sore throat caused by nasogastric tube irritation, the nurse should provide anesthetic lozenges, as prescribed. **(M-S)**

▶ For the first 12 to 24 hours after gastric surgery, stomach contents (obtained by suctioning) are brown. **(M-S)**

▶ During gastric lavage, a nasogastric tube is inserted, the stomach is flushed, and ingested substances are removed through the tube. **(FND)**

▶ After gastric suctioning is discontinued, a patient recovering from a subtotal gastrectomy should receive a clear liquid diet. **(M-S)**

▶ In documenting drainage on a surgical dressing, the nurse should include the size, color, and consistency of the drainage— for example, "10 mm of brown mucoid drainage noted on dressing." **(FND)**

▶ Immunization for hepatitis B should be administered at 0, 1, and 6 months of age. **(PED)**

▶ The classic signs and symptoms of pyloric stenosis are a palpable olive-sized mass (called a pyloric olive) in the right upper quadrant, strong peristaltic movements from left to right during meals, and projectile vomiting. **(PED)**

▶ The preferred site for a permanent colostomy is the descending colon. **(M-S)**

▶ Although rare, arrhythmias and death may result from electroconvulsive therapy. **(PSY)**

▶ A patient who is scheduled for electroconvulsive therapy should receive nothing by mouth after midnight to prevent aspiration while under anesthesia. **(PSY)**

▶ Valvular insufficiency in the veins commonly causes varicosity. **(M-S)**

▶ A patient with a colostomy should restrict fat and fibrous foods and should avoid foods that can obstruct the stoma, such as corn, nuts, and cabbage. **(M-S)**

▶ A patient receiving chemotherapy is placed on reverse isolation because the white blood cell count may be depressed. **(M-S)**

▶ Symptoms of mitral valve stenosis are caused by improper emptying of the left atrium. **(M-S)**

▶ Persistent bleeding after open heart surgery may require protamine sulfate administration to reverse the effects of heparin sodium used during surgery. **(M-S)**

▶ The nurse should teach a patient with heart failure to take digoxin and other drugs as prescribed, restrict sodium intake, restrict fluids as prescribed, get adequate rest, gradually increase walking and other activities, avoid temperature extremes, report signs of heart failure recurrence, and keep regular doctor appointments. **(M-S)**

▶ The nurse should check and maintain the patency of all connections for a chest tube. If an air leak is detected, the nurse should take one Kelly clamp and clamp it near the insertion site. If the bubbling stops, the leak is in the thoracic cavity and the doctor should be notified immediately. If the leak continues, the nurse should take a second clamp and work down the tube until the location of the leak is determined. The nurse should then take appropriate action to stop the leak. **(M-S)**

▶ In two-person cardiopulmonary resuscitation, the rescuers should administer 60 chest compressions per minute and 1 breath for every 5 compressions. **(M-S)**

▶ Mitral valve stenosis can result from rheumatic fever. **(M-S)**

▶ *Atelectasis* refers to incomplete expansion of lung segments or lobules (clusters of alveoli), which may result in lung or lobe collapse. **(M-S)**

▶ The nurse should instruct a patient with an ileal conduit to empty the collection device frequently because the weight of the urine may cause the device to slip from the skin. **(M-S)**

▶ A patient who is receiving cardiopulmonary resuscitation should be placed on a solid, flat surface. **(M-S)**

▶ Brain damage occurs in 4 to 6 minutes after cardiopulmonary function ceases. **(M-S)**

▶ *Climacteric* refers to the transition period during which a woman's reproductive function diminishes and gradually disappears. **(M-S)**

▶ After infratentorial surgery, the patient should be maintained on his side, flat in bed. **(M-S)**

▶ To elicit Babinski's reflex, the nurse strokes the sole of the patient's foot with a moderately sharp object, such as a thumbnail. **(FND)**

▶ In a positive Babinski's reflex, the great toe dorsiflexes and the other toes fan out. **(FND)**

▶ Milk is contraindicated for a patient with an ulcer because its high calcium content stimulates gastric acid secretion. **(M-S)**

▶ When assessing a patient for bladder distention, the nurse should check the contour of the lower abdomen for a rounded mass above the symphysis pubis. **(FND)**

▶ A patient who tests positive for human immunodeficiency virus has been exposed to the virus associated with acquired immunodeficiency syndrome (AIDS) but doesn't necessarily have AIDS. **(M-S)**

▶ A common complication after a prostatectomy is circulatory failure caused by bleeding. **(M-S)**

▶ Most neonates born with human immunodeficiency virus-positive blood develop acquired immunodeficiency syndrome within 4 months. **(PED)**

▶ Because the human immunodeficiency virus (HIV) has been cultured in breast milk, it could be transmitted by an HIV-positive mother who breast-feeds her infant. **(MAT)**

▶ In right-sided heart failure, a major focus of nursing care is decreasing the heart's work load. **(M-S)**

▶ Signs and symptoms of digitalis glycoside toxicity include nausea, vomiting, confusion, and arrhythmias. **(M-S)**

▶ The best way to prevent pressure ulcers is to reposition the bedridden patient at least every 2 hours. **(FND)**

▶ An asthma attack typically begins with wheezing, coughing, and increasing respiratory distress. **(M-S)**

▶ In a patient recovering from a tonsillectomy, frequent swallowing suggests hemorrhage. **(M-S)**

▶ Ileostomies and Hartmann's colostomies are permanent stomas. Loop colostomies and double-barrel colostomies are temporary ones. **(M-S)**

▶ A patient with an ileostomy should eat foods such as spinach and parsley because they act as intestinal tract deodorizers. **(M-S)**

▶ An adrenalectomy can decrease steroid production, which can cause extensive sodium and water loss. **(M-S)**

▶ A fever in the first 24 hours postpartum is most likely caused by dehydration, rather than infection. **(MAT)**

▶ Antiembolism stockings decompress the superficial blood vessels, thereby reducing the risk of thrombus formation. **(FND)**

▶ Before administering morphine sulfate (Duramorph) to a patient suspected of having a myocardial infarction, the nurse should check the patient's respiratory rate. If it is less than 12 breaths/

minute, the nurse should keep emergency equipment readily available for intubation if respiratory depression occurs. **(M-S)**

▶ A patient recovering from supratentorial surgery is normally allowed out of bed 14 to 48 hours after surgery; a patient recovering from infratentorial surgery will be maintained on bed rest for 3 to 5 days. **(M-S)**

▶ Preterm infants or infants who can't maintain a skin temperature of at least 97.6°F (36.4°C) should receive care in an incubator (Isolette) or a radiant warmer. In a radiant warmer, a heat-sensitive probe taped to the infant's skin activates the heater unit automatically to maintain the desired temperature. **(MAT)**

▶ After a patient undergoes femoral-popliteal bypass graft, the nurse must closely monitor peripheral pulses distal to the operative site and circulation. **(M-S)**

▶ After a femoral-popliteal bypass graft, a patient initially should be maintained in semi-Fowler's position to avoid flexion of the graft site. Before discharge, the nurse should instruct the patient to avoid positions that put pressure on the graft site until the next follow-up visit. **(M-S)**

▶ Of the five senses, hearing is the last to be lost in a patient who is entering a coma. **(M-S)**

▶ The most convenient veins for venipuncture in an adult patient are the basilic and median cubital veins in the antecubital space. **(FND)**

▶ Cholelithiasis produces an enlarged, edematous gallbladder with multiple stones and an elevated bilirubin level. **(M-S)**

▶ The antiviral agent zidovudine (Retrovir) has been successful in slowing replication of the human immunodeficiency virus, thereby slowing the development of acquired immunodeficiency syndrome. **(M-S)**

▶ Severe rheumatoid arthritis produces marked edema and congestion, which cause spindle-shaped joints and severe flexion deformities. **(M-S)**

▶ A patient with acquired immunodeficiency syndrome should advise partners of his human immunodeficiency virus status and observe sexual precautions, such as abstinence or condom use.   **(M-S)**

▶ If a radioactive implant becomes dislodged, the nurse should retrieve it with tongs, place it in a lead-shielded container, and notify the radiology department.   **(M-S)**

▶ A patient undergoing radiation therapy should pat the skin dry to avoid abrasions that could easily become infected in an immunocompromised patient.   **(M-S)**

▶ During radiation therapy, a patient should have frequent blood tests, especially white blood cell and platelet counts.   **(M-S)**

▶ The nurse should administer an aluminum hydroxide antacid at least 1 hour after an enteric-coated medication because it can cause premature release of the enteric-coated medication in the stomach.   **(M-S)**

▶ By age 1, an infant has usually tripled its birth weight and can take steps with support.   **(PED)**

▶ *Acid-base balance* refers to the body's hydrogen ion concentration, a measure of the ratio of carbonic acid to bicarbonate ions (1 part carbonic acid to 20 parts bicarbonate is normal).
                                                          (M-S)

▶ Clinical manifestations of amyotrophic lateral sclerosis are progressive atrophy and wasting of muscle groups that eventually affect the respiratory muscles.   **(M-S)**

▶ Metabolic acidosis results from an abnormal loss of bicarbonate ions or excessive production or retention of acid ions.
                                                          (M-S)

▶ *Hemianopia* refers to defective vision or blindness in half the visual field of one or both eyes.   **(M-S)**

▶ Two common manifestations of systemic lupus erythematosus are early-morning joint stiffness and facial erythema in a butterfly pattern.   **(M-S)**

▶ After a total knee replacement, the patient should remain in semi-Fowler's position with the affected leg elevated.   **(M-S)**

▶ When caring for a patient receiving transpyloric feedings, the nurse should monitor for dumping syndrome and hypovolemic shock because the stomach is being bypassed.   **(M-S)**

▶ From 2 to 3 hours before beginning a tube feeding, the nurse should aspirate the patient's stomach contents to verify adequate gastric emptying.   **(FND)**

▶ If a total parenteral nutrition infusion must be interrupted, the nurse should administer dextrose 5% in water at a similar rate because abrupt cessation can result in hypoglycemia.   **(M-S)**

▶ People with type O blood are considered to be universal donors.   **(FND)**

▶ People with type AB blood are considered to be universal recipients.   **(FND)**

▶ In setting-sun sign, which reflects prolonged increased intracranial pressure in children, the eyes are forced downward so that a rim of sclera shows above the irises.   **(PED)**

▶ Intravenous diazepam (Valium) and phenytoin (Dilantin) are used to treat status epilepticus.   **(M-S)**

▶ Disequilibrium syndrome, manifested by nausea, vomiting, restlessness, and twitching, occurs in patients undergoing dialysis and results from a rapid fluid shift.   **(M-S)**

▶ Electroconvulsive therapy usually is used for patients with severe depression that doesn't respond to drug therapy.   **(PSY)**

▶ For electroconvulsive therapy to be effective, the patient usually receives 6 to 12 treatments at a rate of 2 to 3 per week.   **(PSY)**

▶ An indication that spinal shock is resolving is the return of reflex activity in the legs and arms below the level of the injury.   **(M-S)**

▶ Hypovolemia is the most common and fatal complication of severe acute pancreatitis.   **(M-S)**

▶ Oral care for a patient with stomatitis includes mouth rinses with a mixture of equal parts of hydrogen peroxide and water three times daily.   **(M-S)**

▶ *Hertz* (Hz) refers to the unit of measurement of sound frequency.   **(FND)**

▶ In otitis media, the tympanic membrane is bright red and lacks its characteristic light reflex (cone of light).   **(M-S)**

▶ Hearing protection is required when the sound intensity exceeds 84 dB; double hearing protection is required if it exceeds 104 dB.   **(FND)**

▶ In pericardiocentesis, fluid is aspirated from the pericardial sac for analysis or to relieve cardiac tamponade.   **(M-S)**

▶ During labor, the resting phase between contractions should be at least 30 seconds.   **(MAT)**

▶ Urticaria is an early sign of hemolytic transfusion reaction.   **(M-S)**

▶ During peritoneal dialysis, a return of brown dialysate suggests bowel perforation and requires immediate doctor notification.   **(M-S)**

▶ An early sign of ketoacidosis is polyuria, which results from osmotic diuresis.   **(M-S)**

▶ Patients with multiple sclerosis should visually inspect their extremities to ensure proper alignment and freedom from injury.   **(M-S)**

▶ A child with cystic fibrosis should take pancreatic enzyme replacements with meals and snacks.   **(PED)**

▶ Prothrombin, a clotting factor, is produced in the liver.   **(FND)**

▶ Aspirated red bone marrow usually appears rust-red with visible fatty material and white bone fragments.   **(M-S)**

▶ If a patient is menstruating when a urine sample is collected, the nurse should note this on the laboratory slip.   **(FND)**

▶ During lumbar puncture, the nurse must note the initial intracranial pressure and the cerebrospinal fluid color.   **(FND)**

▶ A patient who can't cough to provide a sputum sample for culture may require a heated aerosol treatment to facilitate removal of a sample. **(FND)**

▶ The Dick test detects scarlet fever antigens and immunity or susceptibility to scarlet fever. A positive result indicates no immunity; a negative result indicates immunity. **(M-S)**

▶ The Schick test detects diphtheria antigens and immunity or susceptibility to diphtheria. A positive result indicates no immunity; a negative result indicates immunity. **(M-S)**

▶ The recommended adult dosage of sucralfate (Carafate) for duodenal ulcer is 1 g (one tablet) four times a day 1 hour before meals and at bedtime. **(M-S)**

▶ If eye ointment and eyedrops must be instilled in the same eye, the eyedrops should be instilled first. **(FND)**

▶ When leaving an isolation room, the nurse should remove the gloves before the mask because fewer pathogens are on the mask. **(FND)**

▶ *Lochia rubra* refers to the vaginal discharge of almost pure blood that occurs during the first few days after childbirth. **(MAT)**

▶ *Lochia serosa* refers to the serous vaginal discharge that occurs 4 to 7 days after childbirth. **(MAT)**

▶ *Lochia alba* refers to the vaginal discharge of decreased blood and increased leukocytes that is the final stage of lochia; it occurs 7 to 10 days after childbirth. **(MAT)**

▶ A patient with facial burns or smoke or heat inhalation should be admitted to the hospital for 24-hour observation for delayed tracheal edema. **(M-S)**

▶ In addition to patient teaching, preparation for a colostomy includes withholding oral foods and fluids overnight, performing bowel preparation, and administering a cleansing enema. **(M-S)**

▶ Skeletal traction is applied to a bone using wire pins or tongs. It is the most effective means of traction. **(FND)**

▶ The physiologic changes that take place with burn injuries can be divided into two stages: the hypovolemic stage, during which

intravascular fluid shifts into the interstitial space, and the diuretic stage, during which capillary integrity and intravascular volume are restored, usually 48 to 72 hours after the injury.
(M-S)

▶ The nurse should change total parenteral nutrition tubing every 24 hours and the peripheral intravenous access site dressing every 72 hours. **(M-S)**

▶ The total parenteral nutrition solution should be stored in a refrigerator and removed 30 to 60 minutes before use because delivery of a chilled solution can cause pain, hypothermia, venous spasm, and venous constriction. **(FND)**

▶ *Colostrum* (the precursor of milk) refers to the first secretion from a maternity patient's breasts. **(MAT)**

▶ The length of the uterus increases from 2.6″ (6.5 cm) before pregnancy to 12.8″ (32 cm) at term. **(MAT)**

▶ To estimate the true conjugate (the smallest inlet measurement of the pelvis), deduct 1.5 cm from the diagonal conjugate (usually 12 cm). A true conjugate of 10.5 cm will enable the fetal head (usually 10 cm) to pass. **(MAT)**

▶ The smallest outlet measurement of the pelvis is the intertuberous diameter, which is the transverse diameter between the ischial tuberosities. **(MAT)**

▶ Electronic fetal monitoring is used to assess fetal well-being during labor. If compromised fetal status is suspected, fetal blood pH may be evaluated by obtaining a scalp sample. **(MAT)**

▶ A patient whose carbon monoxide level falls between 20% and 30% should be treated with 100% humidified oxygen. **(M-S)**

▶ When in the room of a patient in isolation for tuberculosis, staff members and visitors should wear ultrafilter masks. **(M-S)**

▶ When providing skin care immediately after pin insertion, the nurse's primary concern is prevention of bone infection. **(M-S)**

▶ A diagnosis of cystic fibrosis is confirmed by a pilocarpine iontophoresis sweat test. Sodium and chloride concentrations of 50 to 60 mEq/L strongly suggest cystic fibrosis. **(PED)**

▶ In a patient who has had an amputation, moist skin may signify venous stasis; dry skin may indicate arterial obstruction. **(M-S)**

▶ Medication isn't routinely injected I.M. into edematous tissue because it may not be absorbed. **(FND)**

▶ In a patient receiving dialysis, an internal shunt is working if the nurse can feel a thrill on palpation or hear a bruit on auscultation. **(M-S)**

▶ In a patient with viral hepatitis, the parenchymal or Kupffer's cells of the liver become severely inflamed, enlarged, and necrotic. **(M-S)**

▶ Early signs of acquired immunodeficiency syndrome include fatigue, night sweats, enlarged lymph nodes, anorexia, weight loss, pallor, and fever. **(M-S)**

▶ When caring for a patient with a radioactive implant, health care workers should stay as far away from the radiation source as possible and should remember the axiom "If you double the distance, you quarter the dose." **(M-S)**

▶ During the manic phase of bipolar affective disorder, nursing care is directed at slowing the patient down because death may result from self-induced exhaustion or injury. **(PSY)**

▶ The nursing care plan for a patient with Alzheimer's disease should focus on safety measures. **(PSY)**

▶ Growth disturbances, such as bone shortening or overgrowth, may occur in children as a result of a fracture of the epiphyseal plate. **(PED)**

▶ In an emergency delivery, enough pressure should be applied to the emerging fetus's head to guide the descent and prevent a rapid change in pressure within the molded fetal skull. **(MAT)**

▶ After delivery, a multiparous woman is more prone to bleeding than a primiparous woman because her uterine muscles may be overstretched and may not contract efficiently. **(MAT)**

▶ Teach a patient with Parkinson's disease to walk using a broad-based gait. **(M-S)**

► The cardinal signs of Parkinson's disease are muscle rigidity, a tremor that begins in the fingers, and akinesia. **(M-S)**

► In a patient with Parkinson's disease, levodopa (Dopar) is prescribed to compensate for the dopamine deficiency. **(M-S)**

► A patient with multiple sclerosis is at increased risk of developing pressure ulcers. **(M-S)**

► Pill-rolling tremor is a classic sign of Parkinson's disease. **(M-S)**

► For a patient with Parkinson's disease, nursing interventions are palliative. **(M-S)**

► Fat embolism, a serious complication of a long bone fracture, produces fever, tachycardia, tachypnea, and anxiety. **(M-S)**

► Metrorrhagia (bleeding between menstrual periods) may be the first sign of cervical cancer. **(M-S)**

► In a rape case, the patient is the primary concern followed by medicolegal considerations. **(PSY)**

► Mannitol is a hypertonic solution and an osmotic diuretic used in the treatment of increased intracranial pressure. **(M-S)**

► When caring for a comatose patient, the nurse should explain each action to the patient in a normal voice. **(FND)**

► When cleaning dentures, the sink should be lined with a washcloth. **(FND)**

► A patient should void within 8 hours after surgery. **(FND)**

► An EEG identifies normal and abnormal brain waves. **(FND)**

► The classic sign of an absence seizure is a vacant facial expression. **(M-S)**

► Migraine headaches are manifested as persistent, severe pain that usually occurs in the temporal region. **(M-S)**

► A patient in a bladder retraining program should be given an opportunity to void every 2 hours during the day and twice at night. **(M-S)**

▶ A decrease in level of consciousness is a cardinal sign of increased intracranial pressure. **(M-S)**

▶ Stool samples for ova and parasite tests should be delivered to the laboratory without delay or refrigeration. **(FND)**

▶ The autonomic nervous system regulates the cardiovascular and respiratory systems. **(FND)**

▶ Ergotamine tartrate (Ergomar) is most effective when taken during the prodromal phase of a migraine or vascular headache. **(M-S)**

▶ Treatment of acute pancreatitis includes nasogastric suctioning to decompress the stomach and meperidine (Demerol) for pain. **(M-S)**

▶ Symptoms of hiatal hernia include a feeling of fullness in the upper abdomen or chest, heartburn, and pain similar to that of angina pectoris. **(M-S)**

▶ The incidence of cholelithiasis is higher in women who have had children than in any other group. **(M-S)**

▶ An acetaminophen (Tylenol) overdose can severely damage the liver. **(M-S)**

▶ The prominent clinical signs of advanced cirrhosis are ascites and jaundice. **(M-S)**

▶ The first symptom of pancreatitis is steady epigastric pain or left upper quadrant pain that radiates from the umbilical area or the back. **(M-S)**

▶ *Somnambulism* is the medical term for sleepwalking. **(M-S)**

▶ Epinephrine (Adrenalin) is a vasoconstrictor. **(M-S)**

▶ An untreated liver laceration or rupture can rapidly progress to hypovolemic shock. **(M-S)**

▶ *Obstipation* refers to extreme, intractable constipation caused by an intestinal obstruction. **(M-S)**

▶ When providing tracheostomy care, the nurse should insert the catheter gently into the tracheostomy tube. When withdrawing the catheter, the nurse should apply intermittent suction for no more than 15 seconds and use a slight twisting motion. **(FND)**

▶ A low-residue diet includes such foods as roasted chicken, rice, and pasta. **(FND)**

▶ A rectal tube should not be inserted for longer than 20 minutes; it can irritate the mucosa of the rectum and cause a loss of sphincter control. **(FND)**

▶ Definitive tests for diagnosing cancer are biopsy and cytologic examination of the specimen. **(M-S)**

▶ Patients in a maintenance program for narcotic abstinence syndrome receive 10 to 40 mg of methadone hydrochloride (Dolophine) in a single daily dose and are monitored to ensure that the medication is ingested. **(PSY)**

▶ Arthrography requires injection of a contrast medium and can identify joint abnormalities. **(M-S)**

▶ Brompton's cocktail is prescribed for patients with terminal cancer to help relieve pain. **(M-S)**

▶ A patient's bed bath should proceed in this order: face, neck, arms, hands, chest, abdomen, back, legs, perineum. **(FND)**

▶ When lifting and moving a patient, the nurse should use the upper leg muscles most to prevent injury. **(FND)**

▶ A sarcoma is a malignant tumor in connective tissue. **(M-S)**

▶ Aluminum hydroxide (Amphojel) neutralizes gastric acid. **(M-S)**

▶ *Subluxation* refers to a partial dislocation or separation with spontaneous reduction of a joint. **(M-S)**

▶ Patient preparation for cholecystography includes ingestion of a contrast medium and a low-fat evening meal. **(FND)**

▶ Barbiturates can cause confusion and delirium in an elderly patient with organic brain disorder. **(M-S)**

▶ In a patient with arthritis, physical therapy is indicated to promote optimal functioning. **(M-S)**

▶ Some patients with hepatitis A may be anicteric (without jaundice) and lack symptoms, but some develop headaches, jaundice, anorexia, fatigue, fever, and respiratory tract infection. **(M-S)**

▶ Hepatitis A won't advance to a carrier state and usually is a milder form of hepatitis. **(M-S)**

▶ During occupied bed changes, the patient should be covered with a bath blanket to promote warmth and prevent exposure. **(FND)**

▶ In the preicteric phase in all forms of hepatitis, the patient is highly contagious. **(M-S)**

▶ Enteric precautions are required for a patient with hepatitis A. **(M-S)**

▶ Cholecystography is ineffective in a patient with jaundice caused by gallbladder disease because the liver cells can't transport the contrast medium to the biliary tract. **(M-S)**

▶ *Anticipatory grief* refers to mourning that occurs for an extended time when one realizes that death is inevitable. **(FND)**

▶ Dehydration is a concern in a patient with diabetes insipidus because this disorder causes polyuria. **(M-S)**

▶ A reducible hernia is one in which the protruding mass spontaneously retracts into the abdomen. **(M-S)**

▶ The following foods can alter stool color: beets (red), cocoa (dark red or brown), licorice (black), spinach (green), and meat protein (dark brown). **(FND)**

▶ Stress management is a short-range goal of psychotherapy. **(PSY)**

▶ The mood most frequently experienced by a patient with organic brain syndrome is irritability. **(PSY)**

▶ Creative intuition is controlled by the right side of the brain. **(PSY)**

▶ Methohexital sodium (Brevital) is the general anesthetic administered to patient scheduled for electroconvulsive therapy. **(PSY)**

▶ When preparing a patient for a skull X-ray, have the patient remove all jewelry and dentures. **(FND)**

▶ The decision to use restraints should be based on the patient's safety needs. **(PSY)**

▶ Diphenhydramine hydrochloride (Benadryl) relieves the extrapyramidal adverse effects of psychotropic medications. **(PSY)**

▶ A patient who is stabilized on lithium (Eskalith) should have blood lithium levels checked 8 to 12 hours after the first dose, then two or three times weekly during the first month. Levels should be checked weekly to monthly during maintenance therapy. **(PSY)**

▶ To prevent purple glove syndrome, the nurse shouldn't administer I.V. phenytoin (Dilantin) through a vein in the back of the hand but should select a larger vessel. **(M-S)**

▶ The primary purpose of psychotropic medications is to decrease the patient's symptoms so that he functions more effectively and is more compliant to therapy. **(PSY)**

▶ Manipulation is considered a maladaptive method of meeting one's needs because it disregards the needs and feelings of others. **(PSY)**

▶ If a patient develops symptoms of lithium toxicity, the nurse should hold one dose and call the doctor. **(PSY)**

▶ A patient taking lithium (Eskalith) for bipolar affective disorder must maintain a balanced diet with adequate salt intake. **(PSY)**

▶ A patient who constantly seeks approval or assistance from staff members and other patients is demonstrating dependent behavior. **(PSY)**

▶ During stage III of surgical anesthesia, unconsciousness occurs and surgery is permitted. **(M-S)**

▶ Alcoholics Anonymous advocates total abstinence. **(PSY)**

▶ Methylphenidate hydrochloride (Ritalin) is the drug of choice for treating attention deficit hyperactivity disorder in children. **(PSY)**

▶ Setting limits is the most effective way to control manipulative behavior. **(PSY)**

▶ Violent outbursts are common in a patient with borderline personality disorder. **(PSY)**

▶ When working with a depressed patient, the nurse should explore meaningful losses. **(PSY)**

▶ An illusion is a misinterpretation of an actual environmental stimulus. **(PSY)**

▶ Anxiety is nonspecific; fear is specific. **(PSY)**

▶ Extrapyramidal adverse effects are common in patients taking antipsychotic medications. **(PSY)**

▶ The nurse should encourage an angry patient to develop a physical exercise program as one of the ways to ventilate feelings. **(PSY)**

▶ Depression is considered clinically significant if it is characterized by exaggerated feelings of sadness, melancholy, dejection, worthlessness, and hopelessness that are inappropriate or out of proportion to reality. **(PSY)**

▶ Free-floating anxiety is anxiousness with generalized apprehension and pessimism for unknown reasons. **(PSY)**

▶ In a patient experiencing intense anxiety, the fight-or-flight reaction (alarm reflex) may take over. **(PSY)**

▶ The fight-or-flight response is a sympathetic nervous system response. **(FND)**

▶ *Confabulation* refers to the use of imaginary experiences or made-up information to fill missing gaps of memory. **(PSY)**

▶ When starting a therapeutic relationship with a patient, the nurse should explain that the purpose of the therapy is to produce a positive change. **(PSY)**

▶ A basic assumption of psychoanalytic theory is that all behavior has meaning.   **(PSY)**

▶ A 6- to 8-month-old infant should be able to sit without assistance.   **(PED)**

▶ Types of regional anesthesia include spinal, caudal, intercostal, epidural, and brachial plexus.   **(M-S)**

▶ Masturbation in prepubescent children and adolescents is considered a normal activity at these developmental stages. **(PED)**

▶ The first step in managing a drug overdose or drug toxicity is to establish and maintain an airway.   **(M-S)**

▶ *Catharsis* refers to the expression of deep feelings and emotions.   **(PSY)**

▶ Respiratory paralysis occurs in stage IV of anesthesia (toxic stage).   **(M-S)**

▶ Neonates delivered by cesarean section have a higher incidence of respiratory distress syndrome.   **(MAT)**

▶ The nurse should suggest ambulation to a postpartal patient who complains of gas pain and flatulence.   **(MAT)**

▶ Massaging the uterus helps stimulate contractions after the placenta is delivered.   **(MAT)**

▶ When providing phototherapy to an infant, the nurse should cover the infant's eyes and genital area.   **(MAT)**

▶ In stage I of anesthesia, consciousness is maintained and is characterized by tranquillity.   **(M-S)**

▶ Dyspnea and sharp, stabbing pain that increases with respiration are symptoms of pleurisy, which can be a complication of pneumonia or tuberculosis.   **(M-S)**

▶ Bronchovesicular breath sounds in peripheral lung fields are abnormal and suggest pneumonia.   **(FND)**

▶ *Wheezing* refers to an abnormal, high-pitched breath sound that is accentuated on expiration.   **(FND)**

▶ Wax or a foreign body in the ear should be gently flushed out by irrigation with warm saline solution. **(FND)**

▶ If a patient complains that his hearing aid is "not working," the nurse should check the switch first to see if it's turned on and then check the batteries. **(FND)**

▶ The nurse should grade hyperactive biceps and triceps reflexes as +4. **(FND)**

▶ Vertigo is the major symptom of a patient with an inner ear infection or disease. **(M-S)**

▶ Loud talking is a sign of hearing impairment. **(M-S)**

▶ A patient with an upper respiratory tract infection should blow the nose with both nostrils open. **(M-S)**

▶ Infants with sickle cell anemia should receive standard well-baby care, including immunizations. **(PED)**

▶ An infant with gastroesophageal reflux should receive formula thickened with cereal. **(PED)**

▶ A patient who has had a cataract removed can begin most normal activities in 3 or 4 days; however, the patient shouldn't bend and lift until a doctor approves these activities. **(M-S)**

▶ If two eye medications are prescribed for twice-daily instillation, they should be administered 5 minutes apart. **(FND)**

▶ Symptoms of corneal transplant rejection include eye irritation and decreasing visual field. **(M-S)**

▶ A child should have a fluoride treatment twice a year. **(PED)**

▶ Wisdom teeth appear between ages 17 and 21. **(PED)**

▶ The narcotic antagonist naloxone (Narcan) may be given to a neonate to correct respiratory depression caused by narcotic administration to the mother during labor. **(MAT)**

▶ Symptoms of respiratory distress syndrome in a neonate include expiratory grunting or whining, sandpaper breath sounds, and seesaw retractions. **(MAT)**

▶ In a postoperative patient, forcing fluids helps prevent constipation. **(FND)**

▶ Cerebral palsy presents as asymmetrical movement, irritability, and excessive feeble crying in a long, thin infant. **(MAT)**

▶ According to the pleasure principle, the psyche seeks pleasure and avoids unpleasant experiences, regardless of the consequences. **(PSY)**

▶ The nurse should assess a breech-birth neonate for hydrocephalus, hematomas, fractures, and other anomalies caused by birth trauma. **(MAT)**

▶ Children ages 3 to 5 don't conceive of death in final terms but do fear separation from parents. **(PED)**

▶ Children ages 5 to 9 view death as a destructive force or, conversely, as an angel coming in the night. They accept death as a final state but don't believe that they are targets. **(PED)**

▶ A conversion disorder allows a patient to resolve a psychological conflict through the loss of a specific physical function—for example, by paralysis, blindness, or inability to swallow. This loss of function is involuntary, but diagnostic tests show no organic cause. **(PSY)**

▶ Graves' disease (hyperthyroidism) is manifested by weight loss, nervousness, dyspnea, palpitations, heat intolerance, increased thirst, exophthalmos (bulging eyes), and goiter. **(M-S)**

▶ When a patient is admitted to the unit in active labor, the nurse's first action is to listen for fetal heart tones. **(MAT)**

▶ In a neonate, long, brittle fingernails are a sign of postmaturity. **(MAT)**

▶ Desquamation (skin peeling) is common in postmature neonates. **(MAT)**

▶ The four types of lipoprotein are chylomicrons (the lowest-density lipoproteins), very-low-density lipoproteins, low-density lipoproteins, and high-density lipoproteins. Health care professionals use cholesterol level fractionation to assess a patient's risk of coronary artery disease. **(M-S)**

▶ Greenstick fractures are the most common fractures in children. **(PED)**

▶ The nurse must administer care in accordance with standards of care established by the American Nurses Association, state regulations, and facility policy. **(FND)**

▶ The *kilocalorie* (kcal) is a unit of energy measurement that represents the amount of heat needed to raise the temperature of 1 kilogram of water 1°C. **(FND)**

▶ A child with measles or chickenpox requires respiratory isolation. **(PED)**

▶ As nutrients move through the body, they undergo ingestion, digestion, absorption, transport, cell metabolism, and excretion. **(FND)**

▶ The body metabolizes alcohol at a fixed rate regardless of serum concentration. **(FND)**

▶ In an alcoholic beverage, its proof reflects its percentage of alcohol multiplied by 2. For example, a 100-proof beverage contains 50% alcohol. **(FND)**

▶ If a patient taking amphotericin B (Fungizone) bladder irrigations for a fungal infection develops systemic candidiasis and must receive I.V. fluconazole (Diflucan), the irrigations can be discontinued because fluconazole covers the bladder infection as well. **(M-S)**

▶ Patients with adult respiratory distress syndrome can have high peak inspiratory pressures. Therefore, the nurse should monitor them closely for signs of spontaneous pneumothorax, such as acute deterioration in oxygenation, absence of breath sounds on the affected side, and crepitus beginning on the affected side. **(M-S)**

▶ Adverse reactions to cyclosporine (Sandimmune) include renal and hepatic toxicity, central nervous system changes (confusion and delirium), GI bleeding, and hypertension. **(M-S)**

▶ *Osteoporosis* refers to a metabolic bone disorder in which the rate of bone resorption exceeds the rate of bone formation. **(M-S)**

▶ The hallmark of ulcerative colitis is recurrent bloody diarrhea, which commonly contains pus and mucus and alternates with asymptomatic remissions. **(M-S)**

▶ Safe sexual practices include massaging, hugging, body rubbing, friendly kissing (dry), masturbating, hand-to-genital touching, wearing a condom, and limiting the numbers of sexual partners. **(M-S)**

▶ Immunosuppressed patients who contract cytomegalovirus (CMV) are at risk for CMV pneumonia and septicemia, which can be fatal. **(M-S)**

▶ A *living will* is a witnessed document that states a patient's desire for certain types of care and treatment, which depends on that patient's wishes and views on quality of life. **(FND)**

▶ The nurse should flush a peripheral heparin lock every 8 hours (if it wasn't used during the previous 8 hours) and as needed with normal saline solution to maintain patency. **(FND)**

▶ Urinary tract infections can produce urinary urgency and frequency, dysuria, abdominal cramps or bladder spasms, and urethral itching. **(M-S)**

▶ A mother should allow her infant to breast-feed until he or she is satisfied. This time may vary from 5 to 20 minutes. **(MAT)**

▶ Mammography is a radiographic technique used to detect breast cysts or tumors, especially those not palpable on physical examination. **(M-S)**

▶ To promote early detection of testicular cancer, palpate the testes during routine physical examinations and encourage the patient to perform monthly self-examinations during a warm shower. **(M-S)**

▶ Quality assurance is a method of determining whether nursing actions and practices meet established standards. **(FND)**

▶ Patients with thalassemia minor require no treatment; those with thalassemia major require frequent transfusions of red blood cells. **(M-S)**

▶ The five rights of medication administration are the right patient, right medication, right dose, right route of administration, and right time. **(FND)**

▶ The purpose of the evaluation phase of the nursing process is to determine whether nursing interventions have enabled the patient to meet desired goals. **(FND)**

▶ Outside of the hospital setting, only the sublingual and translingual forms of nitroglycerin should be used to relieve acute anginal attacks. **(FND)**

▶ The implementation phase of the nursing process involves recording the patient's response to the nursing plan, putting the nursing plan into action, delegating specific nursing interventions, and coordinating the patient's activities. **(FND)**

▶ The Patient's Bill of Rights offers guidance and protection to patients by stating the responsibilities of the hospital and its staff toward patients and their families during hospitalization. **(FND)**

▶ To minimize the omission and distortion of facts, the nurse should record information as soon as it is gathered. **(FND)**

▶ When assessing a patient's health history, the nurse should record the current illness chronologically, beginning with the onset of the problem and continuing to the present. **(FND)**

▶ Chlordiazepoxide (Librium) is the drug of choice for treating alcohol withdrawal symptoms. **(PSY)**

▶ For a patient at risk for alcohol withdrawal, the nurse should assess the pulse rate and blood pressure every 2 hours for the first 12 hours, every 4 hours for the next 24 hours, and every 6 hours thereafter (unless the patient's condition becomes unstable). **(PSY)**

▶ Alcohol detoxification is most successful when carried out in a structured environment by a supportive, nonjudgmental staff. **(PSY)**

▶ A high level of hepatitis B serum marker for 3 months or more after the onset of acute hepatitis B infection suggests the development of chronic hepatitis or a carrier status.   **(M-S)**

▶ Neurogenic bladder dysfunction results from disruption of nerve transmission to the bladder and may be caused by certain spinal cord injuries, diabetes, or multiple sclerosis. **(M-S)**

▶ The nurse should follow these guidelines when caring for a patient who is experiencing alcohol withdrawal: Maintain a calm environment, keep intrusions to a minimum, speak slowly and calmly, adjust lighting to prevent shadows and glare, call the patient by name, and have a friend or family member stay with the patient if possible.   **(PSY)**

▶ The therapeutic regimen for an alcoholic patient includes folic acid, thiamine, and multivitamin supplements as well as adequate food and fluids.   **(PSY)**

▶ A patient addicted to opiates (drugs derived from poppy seeds, such as heroin and morphine) typically experiences withdrawal symptoms within 12 hours after the last dose. The severest symptoms occur within 48 hours and decrease over the next 2 weeks.   **(PSY)**

▶ Oxygen and carbon dioxide move between the lungs and the bloodstream by diffusion.   **(M-S)**

▶ To grade the severity of dyspnea, the nurse may use this system: grade 1, shortness of breath with mild exertion such as walking up steps; grade 2, shortness of breath when walking a short distance at a normal pace on level ground; grade 3, shortness of breath with mild daily activity such as shaving; grade 4, shortness of breath when supine (orthopnea).   **(M-S)**

▶ A patient with Crohn's disease should consume a diet low in residue, fiber, and fat and high in calories, proteins, and carbohydrates and should take vitamin supplements (especially vitamin K).   **(M-S)**

▶ A Logan bar is used postoperatively to prevent suture line strain in a child who has had a cleft lip repair.   **(PED)**

▶ In the three-bottle urine collection method, the patient cleans the meatus and urinates 10 to 15 ml in the first bottle and 15 to 30 ml (midstream) in the second bottle. Then the doctor performs prostatic massage, and the patient voids into the third bottle. **(M-S)**

▶ Findings in the three-bottle urine collection method are interpreted as follows: pus in the urine (pyuria) in the first bottle indicates anterior urethritis; bacteria in the urine in the second bottle indicates bladder infection; bacteria in the third bottle indicates prostatitis. **(M-S)**

▶ Signs and symptoms of aortic stenosis include a loud, rough systolic murmur over the aortic area; exertional dyspnea; fatigue; angina pectoris; arrhythmias; low blood pressure; and emboli. **(M-S)**

▶ Elective surgery is primarily a matter of choice. It isn't essential to the patient's survival, but it may improve the patient's health, comfort, or self-esteem. **(M-S)**

▶ Required surgery is recommended by the doctor. It may be delayed but is inevitable. **(M-S)**

▶ Urgent surgery must be performed within 24 to 48 hours. **(M-S)**

▶ Emergency surgery must be performed immediately. **(M-S)**

▶ Nitrazine paper is used to test the presence of amniotic fluid. **(MAT)**

▶ Drug administration is a dependent activity. The nurse can administer or withhold a drug only with the doctor's permission. **(FND)**

▶ About 85% of arterial emboli originate in the heart chambers. **(M-S)**

▶ Pulmonary embolism usually results from thrombi dislodged from the leg veins. **(M-S)**

▶ The average weight gain during a normal pregnancy is 25 to 30 lb (11.3 to 13.6 kg) total. The patient normally gains 2 to 5 lb (0.9 to 2.3 kg) during the first trimester and slightly less than 1 lb (0.45 kg) per week during the last two trimesters.   **(MAT)**

▶ The nurse shouldn't give false assurance to a patient.   **(FND)**

▶ Neonatal jaundice in the first 24 hours after birth is known as pathological jaundice and is sign of erythroblastosis fetalis.

(MAT)

▶ A classic difference between abruptio placentae and placenta previa is the degree of pain; abruptio placentae produces pain, whereas placenta previa causes painless bleeding.   **(MAT)**

▶ After receiving preoperative medication, a patient isn't competent to sign an informed consent form.   **(FND)**

▶ The conscious interpretation of pain occurs in the cerebral cortex.   **(M-S)**

▶ The dressing on a donor skin graft site shouldn't be disturbed to avoid interfering with new cell growth.   **(M-S)**

▶ A sequela is any abnormal condition that follows and is the result of a disease, a treatment, or an injury.   **(M-S)**

▶ Patient care during sickle cell crisis includes bed rest, oxygen therapy, analgesics as prescribed, I.V. fluid monitoring, and thorough documentation of fluid intake and output.   **(M-S)**

▶ Reactive depression is a response to a specific life event. **(PSY)**

▶ A patient with an ileal conduit should maintain a daily fluid intake of 2,000 ml.   **(M-S)**

▶ The lower central incisors erupt first in an infant at approximately age 4 to 6 months.   **(PED)**

▶ In a closed chest drainage system, continuous bubbling in the water seal chamber or bottle indicates a leak.   **(M-S)**

▶ Palpitation is a sensation of heart pounding or racing associated with normal emotional responses and certain heart disorders.   **(M-S)**

▶ Fat embolism is likely to occur within the first 24 hours after a long-bone fracture. **(M-S)**

▶ Footdrop can occur in a patient with a pelvic fracture because of peroneal nerve compression against the head of the fibula. **(M-S)**

▶ To promote venous return after an amputation, the nurse should wrap an elastic bandage around the distal end of the stump. **(M-S)**

▶ Because a major role of the placenta is to function as a fetal lung, any condition that interrupts normal blood flow to or from the placenta will increase fetal partial pressure of arterial carbon dioxide and decrease fetal pH. **(MAT)**

▶ Water accumulating in the tubing of a ventilator should be removed. **(M-S)**

▶ Precipitate labor lasts for only 3 hours and ends with delivery of the neonate. **(MAT)**

▶ Methylergonovine maleate (Methergine) is an oxytocic agent used to prevent and treat postpartum hemorrhage caused by uterine atony or subinvolution. **(MAT)**

▶ As emergency treatment for excessive uterine bleeding, 0.2 mg of methylergonovine maleate (Methergine) is injected I.V. over 1 minute while the patient's blood pressure and uterine contractions are monitored. **(MAT)**

▶ If a child with a febrile illness is scheduled for an immunization, the immunization should be postponed. **(PED)**

▶ Toilet training should begin when a child shows signs of readiness, such as staying dry for 2 hours or more and verbalizing the urge to urinate. **(PED)**

▶ Most toddlers develop daytime bladder and bowel control between ages 2 and 3 years. (Failure to achieve toilet training by age 5 usually does not indicate pathology but should be investigated by a doctor.) **(PED)**

▶ Projection is the unconscious assigning of a thought, feeling, or action to someone or something else.   **(PSY)**

▶ Sublimation is the channeling of unacceptable impulses into socially acceptable behavior.   **(PSY)**

▶ Repression is an unconscious defense mechanism whereby unacceptable or painful thoughts, impulses, memories, or feelings are pushed from the consciousness or forgotten.   **(PSY)**

▶ The most common administration route for epinephrine is subcutaneous.   **(M-S)**

▶ Hypochondriasis is morbid anxiety about one's health associated with various symptoms not caused by organic disease.   **(PSY)**

▶ Denial is a refusal to acknowledge feelings, thoughts, desires, impulses, or external facts that are consciously intolerable.   **(PSY)**

▶ Reaction formation is the avoidance of anxiety through behavior and attitudes that are the opposite of repressed impulses and drives.   **(PSY)**

▶ Displacement is the transfer of unacceptable feelings to a more acceptable object.   **(PSY)**

▶ Regression is a retreat to an earlier developmental stage. **(PSY)**

▶ The nurse should use Fowler's position for a patient with abdominal pain caused by appendicitis.   **(M-S)**

▶ The nurse shouldn't give analgesics to a patient with abdominal pain caused by appendicitis because these drugs may mask the pain that accompanies a ruptured appendix.   **(M-S)**

▶ As a last-ditch effort, a barbiturate coma may be induced to reverse unrelenting increased intracranial pressure (ICP), which is defined as acute ICP above 40 mm Hg, persistent ICP elevation above 20 mm Hg, or rapidly deteriorating neurologic status.   **(M-S)**

▶ The primary signs and symptoms of epiglottitis are progressive difficulty in swallowing and stridor. **(M-S)**

▶ Salivation is the first step in starch digestion. **(M-S)**

▶ Braxton-Hicks contractions usually are felt in the abdomen and don't cause cervical change, whereas true labor contractions are felt in the front of the abdomen and back and lead to progressive cervical dilation and effacement. **(MAT)**

▶ The average birth weight of neonates born to mothers who smoke is 6 oz (170 g) less than that of neonates born to non-smoking mothers. **(MAT)**

▶ When performing cardiopulmonary resuscitation on an infant, the rescuer should compress the sternum ½″ to 1″ (1.3 to 2.5 cm), using two fingers. **(PED)**

▶ A patient who has a demand pacemaker should measure the pulse rate before rising in the morning, notify the doctor if the pulse rate drops 5 beats/minute, obtain a medical identification card and bracelet, and resume normal activities, including sexual activity. **(M-S)**

▶ Ventricular septal defect occurs because the septum between the left and right ventricles fails to close during the first 8 weeks of gestation. **(PED)**

▶ Transverse colostomy or loop colostomy is a temporary procedure to divert the fecal stream in a patient with acute intestinal obstruction. **(M-S)**

▶ According to Erikson, an older adult (age 65 or older) is in the developmental stage of integrity versus despair. **(PSY)**

▶ Family therapy focuses on the family as a whole rather than the individual. Its major objective is to reestablish rational communication between family members. **(PSY)**

▶ When lifting a patient, a nurse uses the weight of her body instead of the strength in her arms. **(FND)**

▶ Normal values for erythrocyte sedimentation rate range from 0 to 15 mm/hour for men younger than age 50 and from 0 to 20 mm/hour for women younger than age 50. **(M-S)**

▶ A CK-MB level that is more than 5% of total creatine kinase or more than 10 U/L suggests a myocardial infarction. **(M-S)**

▶ Culdoscopy is visualization of the pelvic organs through the posterior vaginal fornix. **(MAT)**

▶ Propranolol (Inderal) blocks sympathetic nerve stimuli that increase cardiac work during exercise or stress, which reduces heart rate, blood pressure, and myocardial oxygen consumption. **(M-S)**

▶ After a myocardial infarction, electrocardiogram changes (ST-segment elevation, T-wave inversion, and Q-wave enlargement) usually appear in the first 24 hours but may not appear until the 5th or 6th day. **(M-S)**

▶ Cardiogenic shock is manifested by systolic blood pressure below 80 mm Hg, gray skin, diaphoresis, cyanosis, weak pulse rate, tachycardia or bradycardia, and oliguria of less than 30 ml/hour of urine. **(M-S)**

▶ A patient on a low-sodium diet shouldn't eat foods such as cottage cheese, fish, canned beans, chuck steak, chocolate pudding, Italian salad dressing, dill pickles, and beef broth. **(M-S)**

▶ High-potassium foods include dried prunes, watermelon (15.3 mEq/portion), dried lima beans (14.5 mEq/portion), soybeans, bananas, and oranges. **(M-S)**

▶ A nurse may clarify a doctor's explanation to a patient about an operation or a procedure but must refer questions about informed consent to the doctor. **(FND)**

▶ When caring for a hostile or angry patient, the nurse should attempt to remain calm, listen without showing disapproval, use short sentences, and speak in a firm, quiet voice. **(PSY)**

▶ A sick or injured child with limited communication skills may be able to express feelings or concerns by drawing a picture with crayons or markers. **(PED)**

▶ When obtaining a health history from an acutely ill or agitated patient, the nurse should limit questions to those that provide necessary information. **(FND)**

▶ If a chest drainage system line is broken or interrupted, the nurse should immediately clamp the tube. **(FND)**

▶ The nurse shouldn't use her thumb to take a patient's pulse rate because the thumb has a pulse of its own and may be confused with the patient's pulse. **(FND)**

▶ An inspiration and an expiration count as one respiration. **(FND)**

▶ Kussmaul's respirations are faster and deeper than normal respirations and occur without pauses, as in diabetic ketoacidosis. **(M-S)**

▶ Cheyne-Stokes respirations are characterized by alternating periods of apnea and deep, rapid breathing as seen in central nervous system disorders. **(M-S)**

▶ Hyperventilation can result from an increased frequency of breathing, an increased tidal volume, or both. **(M-S)**

▶ Apnea is the absence of spontaneous respirations. **(M-S)**

▶ Before a thyroidectomy, a patient may receive potassium iodide, antithyroid drugs, and propranolol (Inderal) to prevent thyroid storm during surgery. **(M-S)**

▶ Normal respirations are known as eupnea. **(FND)**

▶ During a blood pressure measurement, the patient should rest the arm against a surface because using muscle strength to hold up the arm may raise the blood pressure. **(FND)**

▶ Major unalterable risk factors for coronary artery disease include heredity, sex, race, and age. **(FND)**

▶ The nurse should teach a pregnant vegetarian to obtain protein from alternative sources, such as nuts, soybeans, and legumes. **(MAT)**

▶ Inspection is the most frequently used assessment technique. **(FND)**

▶ The nurse should instruct a pregnant patient to take only prescribed prenatal vitamins because over-the-counter megavitamins may harm the fetus. **(MAT)**

▶ High-sodium foods can cause fluid retention, especially in pregnant patients. **(MAT)**

▶ A pregnant patient can avoid constipation and hemorrhoids by adding fiber to her diet. **(MAT)**

▶ The normal life span of red blood cells (erythrocytes) is 110 to 120 days. **(M-S)**

▶ Ritualism and negativism are typical toddler behaviors. They occur during the developmental stage identified by Erikson as autonomy versus shame and doubt. **(PSY)**

▶ Accidents are the leading cause of death in children and usually are age-related—for example, toddlers are injured in falls and teenagers are injured in sports. **(PED)**

▶ Urinary tract infections are more common in girls and women than in boys and men because the shorter urethra in the female urinary tract makes the bladder more accessible to bacteria, especially *Escherichia coli*. **(M-S)**

▶ Visual acuity of 20/100 means that the patient sees at 20′ (6 m) what a person with normal vision sees at 100′ (30 m). **(M-S)**

▶ According to Freud, the oral stage occurs between birth and age 18 months. **(PED)**

▶ Penicillin should be administered orally 1 to 2 hours before meals or 2 to 3 hours after meals because food may interfere with the drug's absorption. **(M-S)**

▶ For an infant, the nurse should start an I.V. line in a peripheral vein or a vein in the temporal region. **(PED)**

▶ Mild reactions to local anesthetics may include palpitations, tinnitus, vertigo, apprehension, confusion, and a metallic taste in the mouth. **(M-S)**

▶ When administering an oral medication to a toddler, the nurse should have the child place the medication on the back of the tongue and swallow it with fruit juice or water. **(PED)**

▶ Family members of an elderly person in a long-term care facility should transfer some personal items (such as photographs, a favorite chair, and knickknacks) to the person's room to provide a homey atmosphere. **(FND)**

▶ About 22% of cardiac output goes to the kidneys. **(M-S)**

▶ To ensure accurate central venous pressure readings, the nurse should place the manometer or transducer level with the phlebostatic axis. **(M-S)**

▶ A patient who has lost 2,000 to 2,500 ml of blood will have a pulse rate of 140 beats/minute (or higher), display a systolic blood pressure of 50 to 60 mm Hg, and appear confused and lethargic. **(M-S)**

▶ Arterial bleeding is bright red, flows rapidly, and (because it is pumped directly from the heart) spurts with each heartbeat.
(M-S)

▶ Venous blood is dark red and tends to ooze from a wound.
(M-S)

▶ Orthostatic blood pressure is taken with the patient in the supine, sitting, and standing positions and with 1 minute between each reading. A 10-mm Hg decrease in blood pressure or a pulse rate increase of 10 beats/minute suggests volume depletion. **(M-S)**

▶ Pulsus alternans is a regular pulse rhythm with alternating weak and strong beats. It occurs in ventricular enlargement because the stroke volume varies with each heartbeat. **(FND)**

▶ A pneumatic antishock garment should be used cautiously with pregnant women and patients with head injuries.   **(M-S)**

▶ After a patient's circulating volume has been restored, the nurse should remove the pneumatic antishock garment gradually, starting with the abdominal chamber and followed by each leg. Removal should be done under a doctor's supervision.   **(M-S)**

▶ Most hemolytic transfusion reactions associated with the mismatching of ABO blood types stem from identification number errors.   **(M-S)**

▶ Circumstantiality is a disturbance in associated thought and speech patterns in which a patient gives unnecessary, minute details and digresses into inappropriate thoughts, which delay communication of central ideas or goal achievement.   **(PSY)**

▶ Warming of blood above 107° F (41.7° C) can cause hemolysis.   **(M-S)**

▶ Cardiac output is the amount of blood ejected from the heart each minute and is expressed in liters per minute.   **(M-S)**

▶ Stroke volume is the volume of blood ejected from the heart during systole.   **(M-S)**

▶ Total parenteral nutrition solution contains dextrose, amino acids, and additives, such as electrolytes, minerals, and vitamins.   **(M-S)**

▶ The most common type of neurogenic shock is spinal shock. It usually occurs 30 to 60 minutes after a spinal cord injury.   **(M-S)**

▶ After a spinal cord injury, peristalsis stops within 24 hours and usually returns within 3 to 4 days.   **(M-S)**

▶ Toxic shock syndrome is manifested by a temperature of at least 102° F (38.8° C), an erythematous rash, and systolic blood pressure below 90 mm Hg. From 1 to 2 weeks after the onset of these signs, desquamation (especially on the palms and soles) occurs.   **(M-S)**

▶ The signs and symptoms of anaphylaxis commonly are caused by histamine release. **(M-S)**

▶ The most common cause of septic shock is gram-negative bacteria, such as *Escherichia coli*, *Klebsiella*, and *Pseudomonas* organisms. **(M-S)**

▶ Bruits are vascular sounds that resemble heart murmurs and result from turbulent blood flow through a diseased or partially obstructed artery. **(M-S)**

▶ Urine pH normally ranges from 4.5 to 8.0. **(M-S)**

▶ Urine pH greater than 8.0 can result from a urinary tract infection, high-alkali diet, or systemic alkalosis. **(M-S)**

▶ Urine pH less than 4.5 may indicate a high-protein diet, fever, or metabolic acidosis. **(M-S)**

▶ Before a percutaneous renal biopsy, the patient should be placed on a firm surface and positioned on the abdomen with a sandbag under the abdomen to stabilize the kidneys. **(M-S)**

▶ Nephrotic syndrome is characterized by marked proteinuria, hypoalbuminemia, mild to severe dependent edema, ascites, and weight gain. **(M-S)**

▶ Underwater exercise is a form of therapy performed in a Hubbard tank. **(M-S)**

▶ Most women with trichomoniasis have a malodorous, frothy, greenish gray vaginal discharge; other women may have no signs or symptoms. **(M-S)**

▶ Voiding cystourethrography may be done to detect bladder and urethral abnormalities. In this test, contrast medium is instilled by gentle syringe pressure through a urethral catheter, and overhead X-ray films are taken to visualize bladder filling and excretion. **(M-S)**

▶ Cystourethrography may be done to help identify the cause of urinary tract infections, congenital anomalies, and incontinence. It also is used to assess for prostate lobe hypertrophy in men. **(M-S)**

▶ Herpes simplex, characterized by recurrent episodes of blisters on the skin and mucous membranes, has two variations. In Type 1, the blisters appear in the nasolabial region; in Type 2, they appear on the genitals, anus, buttocks, and thighs. **(M-S)**

▶ Most patients with *Chlamydia trachomatis* infection are asymptomatic, but some develop an inflamed urethral meatus, dysuria, and urinary urgency and frequency. **(M-S)**

▶ The hypothalamus regulates the autonomic nervous system and endocrine functions. **(M-S)**

▶ If a fetus develops late deceleration (a sign of fetal hypoxia), the nurse should instruct the mother to lie on her left side and then should administer 8 to 10 L of oxygen per minute by mask or cannula. The nurse should notify the doctor. (The side-lying position removes pressure on the inferior vena cava.) **(MAT)**

▶ Oxytocin (Pitocin) promotes lactation and uterine contractions. **(MAT)**

▶ The upper respiratory tract warms and humidifies inspired air and plays a role in taste, smell, and mastication. **(FND)**

▶ A patient whose chest excursion is less than normal (3″ to 6″ [7.5 to 15 cm]) must use accessory muscles to breathe. **(M-S)**

▶ Signs of accessory muscle use include shoulder elevation, intercostal muscle retraction, and scalene and sternocleidomastoid muscle use during respiration. **(FND)**

▶ Lanugo covers the fetus's body until about 20 weeks' gestation. Then it begins to disappear from the face, trunk, arms, and legs, in that order. **(MAT)**

▶ Although a cleft palate can be repaired at any time, the optimal time for corrective surgery is before the child begins speaking and learns faulty speech habits. **(PED)**

▶ In a neonate, hypoglycemia is manifested by temperature instability, hypotonia, jitteriness, and seizures. Premature, postmature, small-for-gestational-age, and large-for-gestational-age neonates are prone to this disorder. **(MAT)**

▶ An infant with a gastrostomy tube should receive a pacifier during feeding unless contraindicated to allow normal sucking activity and satisfy oral needs. **(PED)**

▶ Signs and symptoms of toxicity from thyroid replacement therapy include rapid pulse rate, diaphoresis, irritability, weight loss, dysuria, and sleep disturbance. **(M-S)**

▶ The most common allergic reaction to penicillin is a rash. **(M-S)**

▶ An early sign of aspirin toxicity is deep, rapid respirations. **(M-S)**

▶ The most serious and irreversible consequence of lead poisoning is mental retardation, which results from neurologic damage. **(M-S)**

▶ Treatment for Legg-Calvé-Perthes disease consists of restricting weight bearing and using a device such as an abduction brace or a harness sling to protect the affected joint while revascularization and bone healing occur. **(PED)**

▶ To assess dehydration in the adult, the nurse should check skin turgor on the sternum. **(M-S)**

▶ Legg-Calvé-Perthes disease (also known as coxa plana) is manifested in aseptic necrosis of the head of the femur. **(PED)**

▶ In developing a diet for a patient with a peptic ulcer, the nurse should remember this guideline: The type of diet is less important than including foods in the diet that the patient can tolerate. **(M-S)**

▶ A patient with a colostomy needs to establish an irrigation schedule so that regular emptying of the bowel occurs without stomal discharge between irrigations. **(M-S)**

▶ Idea of reference is an incorrect belief that the statements or actions of others are related to oneself. **(PSY)**

▶ When using rotating tourniquets, the nurse shouldn't restrict the blood supply to an arm or a leg for more than 45 minutes at a time. **(M-S)**

▶ A patient with diabetes should eat high-fiber foods because they blunt the rise in glucose level that normally follows a meal. **(M-S)**

▶ Jugular vein distention occurs in heart failure because the left ventricle can't empty the heart of blood as fast as blood enters from the right ventricle, resulting in congestion in the entire venous system. **(M-S)**

▶ When patients use axillary crutches, their palms should bear the brunt of the weight. **(FND)**

▶ The leading causes of blindness in the United States are diabetes mellitus and glaucoma. **(M-S)**

▶ After a thyroidectomy, the patient should remain in semi-Fowler's position with the head neither hyperextended nor hyperflexed to avoid pressure on the suture line. This can be accomplished by a cervical pillow. **(M-S)**

▶ Premenstrual syndrome may cause abdominal distention, engorged and painful breasts, backache, headache, nervousness, irritability, restlessness, and tremors. **(M-S)**

▶ Treatment of dehiscence (pathologic opening of a wound) consists of covering the wound with a moist sterile dressing and notifying the doctor. **(M-S)**

▶ When a patient has a radical mastectomy, the ovaries also may be removed because they are a source of estrogen, which stimulates tumor growth. **(M-S)**

▶ Atropine sulfate blocks the effects of acetylcholine, thereby obstructing its vagal effects on the sinoatrial node and increasing heart rate. **(M-S)**

▶ Activities of daily living include eating, bathing, dressing, grooming, toileting, and interacting socially. **(FND)**

▶ Salicylates, particularly aspirin, are the treatment of choice in rheumatoid arthritis because they decrease inflammation and relieve joint pain. **(M-S)**

▶ Deep, intense pain that usually worsens at night and is unrelated to movement suggests bone pain. **(M-S)**

▶ Pain that follows prolonged or excessive exercise and subsides with rest suggests muscle pain. **(M-S)**

▶ Normal gait has two phases: the stance phase, in which the patient's foot rests on the ground, and the swing phase, in which the patient's foot moves forward. **(FND)**

▶ The major hemodynamic changes associated with cardiogenic shock are decreased left ventricular function and decreased cardiac output. **(M-S)**

▶ Before thyroidectomy, the patient should be advised that he may experience hoarseness or loss of the voice for several days after surgery. **(M-S)**

▶ Acceptable adverse effects of long-term steroid use include weight gain, acne, headaches, fatigue, and increased urine retention. **(M-S)**

▶ Unacceptable adverse effects of long-term steroid use are dizziness on rising, nausea, vomiting, thirst, and pain. **(M-S)**

▶ After a craniotomy, nursing care includes maintaining normal intracranial pressure, maintaining cerebral perfusion pressure, and preventing injury related to cerebral and cellular ischemia. **(M-S)**

▶ Neonates typically need to consume 50 to 55 cal/lb of body weight daily. **(MAT)**

▶ Folic acid and vitamin B_{12} are essential for nucleoprotein synthesis and red blood cell maturation. **(M-S)**

▶ Immediately after intracranial surgery, nursing care includes not giving the patient anything by mouth until gag and cough reflexes return, monitoring vital signs and assessing level of consciousness (LOC) for signs of increasing intracranial pressure, and giving analgesics that don't mask the patient's LOC. **(M-S)**

▶ Chest physiotherapy includes postural drainage, chest percussion and vibration, coughing, and deep-breathing exercises.
(M-S)

▶ The nurse should encourage parents to communicate with their hearing-impaired child through mime, gestures, and body language. **(PED)**

▶ Kawasaki disease is characterized by a high temperature for 5 or more days, strawberry tongue, red and dry lips, cervical lymphadenopathy, carditis, hand edema, rash on the soles or palms, and bilateral congestion of the ocular conjunctivae. **(PED)**

▶ Cushing's syndrome results from excessive levels of adrenocortical hormones and is manifested by fat pads on the face (moon face) and over the upper back (buffalo hump), acne, mood swings, hirsutism, amenorrhea, and decreased libido. **(M-S)**

▶ When discontinuing long-term prednisone (Deltasone) therapy, the nurse should taper the dose slowly to allow for monitoring of disease flare-ups and for the return of hypothalamic-pituitary-adrenal function in order to prevent an Addison-like crisis. **(M-S)**

▶ Pulsus paradoxus (a pulse that becomes weak during inspiration and strong during expiration) may be a sign of cardiac tamponade. **(M-S)**

▶ Substances expelled through portals of exit include saliva, mucus, feces, urine, vomitus, blood, and vaginal and penile discharge. **(M-S)**

▶ A microorganism may be transmitted directly by contact with an infected body or droplets or indirectly by contact with contaminated air, soil, water, or fluids. **(M-S)**

▶ A postmenopausal woman receiving estrogen therapy is at increased risk for developing gallbladder disease and breast cancer. **(M-S)**

▶ The approximate oxygen concentrations delivered by nasal cannula are as follows: 1 L = 24%, 2 L = 28%, 3 L = 32%, 4 L= 36%, and 5 L = 40%. **(M-S)**

▶ Because oxytocin (Pitocin) stimulates powerful uterine contractions during labor, it must be administered under close observation to help prevent maternal and fetal distress. **(MAT)**

▶ Cardinal features of diabetes insipidus include polydipsia (excessive thirst) and polyuria (increased urination to 5 L/24 hours). **(M-S)**

▶ A patient with low specific gravity (1.001 to 1.005) may have an increased desire for cold water. **(M-S)**

▶ Diabetic coma can occur when the blood glucose level drops below 60 mg/dl. **(M-S)**

▶ For a patient with heart failure, the nurse should elevate the head of the bed 8″ to 12″ (20 to 30 cm), provide a bedside commode, and administer digitalis glycosides and diuretics as prescribed. **(M-S)**

▶ Group therapy provides an opportunity for each group member to examine interactions, learn and practice successful interpersonal communication skills, and explore emotional conflicts. **(PSY)**

▶ The primary reason for treating streptococcal sore throat with antibiotics is to protect the heart valves and prevent rheumatic fever. **(M-S)**

▶ A patient with a nasal fracture may lose consciousness during reduction. **(M-S)**

▶ Hoarseness and change in voice is usually the first sign of laryngeal cancer. **(M-S)**

▶ The lungs, colon, and rectum are among the most common cancer sites. **(M-S)**

▶ The most common preoperative problem in elderly patients is lower-than-normal total blood volume. **(M-S)**

▶ Mannitol (Osmitrol), an osmotic diuretic, is administered to reduce intraocular or intracranial pressure. **(M-S)**

▶ When a cerebrovascular accident is suspected, the nurse should place the patient on the affected side to promote lung expansion on the unaffected side. **(M-S)**

▶ For a patient who has had chest surgery, the nurse should recommend sitting upright and performing deep-breathing and coughing exercises. These actions promote lung expansion, secretion removal, and optimal pulmonary functioning. **(M-S)**

▶ During fetal heart monitoring, variable deceleration indicates umbilical cord compression or prolapse. **(MAT)**

▶ During every sleep cycle, the sleeper passes through four stages of nonrapid-eye-movement sleep and one stage of rapid-eye-movement sleep. **(M-S)**

▶ The phases of mitosis are prophase, metaphase, anaphase, and telophase. **(FND)**

▶ Korsakoff's syndrome is believed to be a chronic form of Wernicke's encephalopathy marked by hallucinations, confabulation, amnesia, and disturbances of orientation. **(PSY)**

▶ A patient taking calcifediol (Calderol) should avoid concomitant use of preparations that contain vitamin D. **(M-S)**

▶ A patient should begin and end a 24-hour urine collection period with an empty bladder. (For example, if the doctor orders urine to be collected from 0800 Thursday to 0800 Friday, the urine voided at 0800 Thursday should be discarded and the urine voided at 0800 Friday should be retained.) **(M-S)**

▶ In a patient receiving digoxin (Lanoxin), a low potassium level increases the risk of digitalis toxicity. **(M-S)**

▶ Blood urea nitrogen values normally range from 10 to 20 mg/dl. **(M-S)**

▶ Flurazepam (Dalmane) toxicity is manifested by confusion, hallucinations, and ataxia. **(M-S)**

▶ A silent myocardial infarction is one that produces no symptoms. **(M-S)**

▶ Adverse reactions to verapamil (Isoptin) include dizziness, headache, constipation, hypotension, and atrioventricular conduction disturbances. The drug also may increase the serum digoxin level. **(M-S)**

▶ When a rectal tube is used to relieve flatulence or enhance peristalsis, it should be inserted for no more than 20 minutes. **(M-S)**

▶ Yellowish green discharge on a wound dressing indicates infection and should be cultured. **(M-S)**

▶ Sickle cell crisis can cause severe abdominal, thoracic, muscular, and bone pain along with painful swelling of soft tissue in the hands and feet. **(M-S)**

▶ Oral candidiasis (thrush) is characterized by cream-colored or bluish white patches on the oral mucous membrane. **(M-S)**

▶ Treatment for a patient with cystic fibrosis may include drug therapy, exercises to improve breathing and posture and facilitate mobilization of pulmonary secretions, a high-salt diet, and pancreatic enzyme supplements with snacks and meals. **(M-S)**

▶ After surgical reconstruction of an imperforate anus and formation of a temporary colostomy, an infant should remain prone with the hips elevated. **(PED)**

▶ A patient with antisocial personality disorder frequently engages in confrontations with authority figures, such as police, parents, and school officials. **(PSY)**

▶ A patient with paranoid personality disorder exhibits suspicion, hypervigilance, and hostility toward others. **(PSY)**

▶ Child neglect consists of abandonment or failure to provide a safe, secure environment for a child. **(PED)**

▶ Depression is the most common psychiatric disorder. **(PSY)**

▶ Cytomegalovirus is the leading cause of congenital viral infections. **(MAT)**

▶ Most infants with cerebral palsy are long and thin, move asymmetrically, have difficulty feeding, and cry excessively or feebly.
(PED)

▶ Pancreatic cancer may cause weight loss, jaundice, and intermittent dull-to-severe epigastric pain.   **(M-S)**

▶ Adverse reactions to tricyclic antidepressant drugs include tachycardia, orthostatic hypotension, hypomania, lowered seizure threshold, tremors, weight gain, problems with erections or orgasms, and anxiety.   **(PSY)**

▶ The nurse should follow standard precautions in the routine care of all patients.   **(FND)**

▶ Metastasis is the spread of cancer from one organ or body part to another through the lymphatic system, circulation system, or cerebrospinal fluid.   **(M-S)**

▶ Tocolytic therapy is indicated in premature labor but contraindicated in fetal death, fetal distress, or severe hemorrhage.
(MAT)

▶ The management of pulmonary edema focuses on opening the airways, supporting ventilation and perfusion, improving cardiac functioning, reducing preload, and reducing patient anxiety.
(M-S)

▶ Factors that contribute to the death of patients with Alzheimer's disease include infection, malnutrition, and dehydration. **(M-S)**

▶ Hodgkin's disease is characterized by painless, progressive enlargement of cervical lymph nodes and other lymphoid tissue resulting from proliferation of Reed-Sternberg cells, histiocytes, and eosinophils.   **(M-S)**

▶ Huntington's disease (chorea) is a hereditary disease characterized by degeneration in the cerebral cortex and basal ganglia.
(M-S)

▶ A patient with Huntington's disease may exhibit suicidal ideation.   **(M-S)**

▶ At discharge, an amputee should be able to demonstrate proper stump care and perform stump-toughening exercises. **(M-S)**

▶ Acute tubular necrosis is the most common cause of acute renal failure. **(M-S)**

▶ Common complications of ice water lavage are vomiting and aspiration. **(M-S)**

▶ Foods high in vitamin D include fortified milk, fish, liver, liver oil, herring, and egg yolk. **(M-S)**

▶ Through ultrasonography, the biophysical profile assesses fetal well-being by measuring fetal breathing movements, gross body movements, fetal tone, reactive fetal heart rate (nonstress test), and qualitative amniotic fluid volume. **(MAT)**

▶ For a pelvic examination, the patient should be in the lithotomy position with her buttocks extending 2½" (6.4 cm) past the end of the examination table. **(M-S)**

▶ If a patient can't assume a lithotomy position, she may lie on her left side. **(M-S)**

▶ A male examiner should have a female assistant present during a vaginal examination for the patient's emotional comfort and the examiner's legal protection. **(M-S)**

▶ Cervical secretions are clear and stretchy before ovulation and white and opaque after ovulation. They normally are odorless and don't irritate the mucosa. **(M-S)**

▶ A neonate whose mother has diabetes should be assessed for hyperinsulinism. **(MAT)**

▶ Epigastric pain is a late symptom in a patient with preeclampsia and requires immediate medical intervention. **(MAT)**

▶ After a stillbirth, the mother should be allowed to hold the neonate to help her come to terms with the death. **(MAT)**

▶ The concept of object permanence develops between ages 6 and 8 months. **(PED)**

▶ A child begins to understand cause-and-effect relations at age 2 years, during the sensorimotor stage. **(PED)**

▶ Attention deficit hyperactivity disorder and learning disabilities are more common among boys than girls. **(PED)**

▶ A patient with an ileostomy shouldn't eat corn because it may obstruct the pouch opening. **(M-S)**

▶ Molding describes the process by which the fetal head changes shape to facilitate movement through the birth canal. **(MAT)**

▶ Liver dysfunction affects the metabolism of certain drugs. **(M-S)**

▶ If a patient receives a pudendal block before delivery, the nurse should monitor the patient's blood pressure closely. **(MAT)**

▶ If a patient suddenly becomes hypotensive during labor, the nurse should increase the infusion rate of I.V. fluids, as prescribed. **(MAT)**

▶ The best technique for assessing jaundice in a neonate is to blanch the tip of the nose or the area just above the umbilicus. **(MAT)**

▶ During fetal heart monitoring, early deceleration is caused by head compression during labor. **(MAT)**

▶ After the placenta is delivered, the nurse may add oxytocin (Pitocin) to the patient's I.V. solution as prescribed to promote postpartum involution of the uterus and stimulate lactation. **(MAT)**

▶ Pica is a craving to eat nonfood items, such as dirt, crayons, chalk, glue, starch, or hair. It may occur during pregnancy and can endanger the fetus. **(M-S)**

▶ A pregnant patient should take folic acid because this nutrient is required for rapid cell division. **(MAT)**

▶ Edema that accompanies burns and malnutrition is caused by decreased capillary osmotic pressure. **(M-S)**

▶ Hyponatremia is most likely to occur as a complication of nasogastric suctioning. **(M-S)**

▶ For a man who suffers complete spinal cord separation at S4, erection and ejaculation aren't possible. **(M-S)**

▶ The early signs of pulmonary edema—dyspnea on exertion and coughing—reflect interstitial fluid accumulation and diminished ventilation and alveolar perfusion. **(M-S)**

▶ Methylprednisolone sodium succinate (Solu-Medrol) is a first-line drug used to control edema after spinal cord trauma. **(M-S)**

▶ For the patient who is recovering from an intracranial bleed, the nurse should maintain a quiet, restful environment for the first few days. **(M-S)**

▶ The patient taking clomiphene citrate (Clomid) to induce ovulation should be informed of the possibility of multiple births with this drug. **(MAT)**

▶ Neurosyphilis is associated with widespread central nervous system damage, including general paresis, personality changes, slapping gait, and blindness. **(M-S)**

▶ A woman who has sustained a spinal cord injury can still become pregnant. **(M-S)**

▶ In a patient who has had a cerebrovascular accident, the most serious complication is increasing intracranial pressure. **(M-S)**

▶ If needed, cervical suturing usually is done between 14 and 18 weeks' gestation to reinforce an incompetent cervix and maintain pregnancy. Such suturing typically is removed by 35 weeks' gestation. **(MAT)**

▶ A patient with an intracranial hemorrhage should undergo arteriography to determine the site of the bleeding. **(M-S)**

▶ Factors that affect drug action include absorption, distribution, metabolism, and excretion. **(M-S)**

▶ During the first trimester, a pregnant woman should avoid all medications unless doing so would adversely affect her health.
(MAT)

▶ Before prescribing a medication for a woman of childbearing age, the prescriber should ask for the date of her last menstrual period and ask if she may be pregnant. **(M-S)**

▶ Most medications a breast-feeding mother takes appear in breast milk. **(MAT)**

▶ Acidosis may cause insulin resistance. **(M-S)**

▶ A patient with glucose-6-phosphate dehydrogenase deficiency may develop acute hemolytic anemia when given a sulfonamide. **(M-S)**

▶ The Food and Drug Administration has established five categories of drugs based on their potential for causing birth defects: A — No evidence of risk; B — No risk found in animals, but no studies have been done in women; C — Animal studies have shown an adverse effect, but the drug may be beneficial to women despite the potential risk; D — Evidence of risk, but its benefits may outweigh its risks; and X — Fetal anomalies noted, and the risks clearly outweigh the potential benefits. **(MAT)**

▶ The five basic activities of the digestive system include ingestion, movement of food, digestion, absorption, and defecation. **(M-S)**

▶ The nurse should use the bell of the stethoscope to listen for venous hums and cardiac murmurs. **(FND)**

▶ Signs and symptoms of acute pancreatitis include epigastric pain, vomiting, bluish discoloration of the left flank (Grey Turner's sign), bluish discoloration of the periumbilical area (Cullen's sign), low-grade fever, tachycardia, and hypotension. **(M-S)**

▶ A patient with a gastric ulcer may complain of gnawing or burning epigastric pain. **(M-S)**

▶ The nurse can assess a patient's general knowledge by asking questions such as "Who is the president of the United States?" **(FND)**

▶ To test the first cranial nerve (olfactory nerve), the nurse should ask the patient to close the eyes, occlude one nostril, and identify a nonirritating substance (such as peppermint or cinnamon) by smell. Then the nurse should repeat the test with the patient's other nostril occluded. **(M-S)**

▶ Salk and Sabin introduced the oral polio vaccine. **(M-S)**

▶ A patient with a disease of the cerebellum or posterior column has an ataxic gait, characterized by staggering, unsteadiness, and an inability to remain steady when standing with the feet together. **(M-S)**

▶ Improved outcomes for trauma patients are directly related to early resuscitation, aggressive management of shock, and appropriate definitive care. **(M-S)**

▶ To check for cerebrospinal fluid leakage, the nurse should inspect the patient's nose and ears. If the patient can sit up, the nurse should observe for leakage as the patient leans forward. **(M-S)**

▶ For a child suspected of having Reye's syndrome, the nurse should ask the parents if the child received aspirin during the current or a recent illness. **(PED)**

▶ "Locked-in" syndrome is complete paralysis caused by brain stem damage; only the eyes can be moved voluntarily. **(M-S)**

▶ Neck dissection, the surgical removal of the cervical lymph nodes, is performed to prevent the spread of malignant head and neck tumors. **(M-S)**

▶ A patient with cholecystitis typically complains of right epigastric pain, which may radiate to the right scapula or shoulder; nausea; and vomiting, especially after eating a heavy meal. **(M-S)**

▶ A patient with a ruptured ectopic pregnancy commonly has sharp lower abdominal pain with spotting and cramping and may experience abdominal rigidity, rapid and shallow respirations, tachycardia, and shock. **(MAT)**

▶ Atropine is used preoperatively to reduce secretions. **(M-S)**

▶ Serum calcium levels normally range from 4.5 to 5.5 mEq/L (8.0 to 10.5 mg/dl). **(M-S)**

▶ Suppressor T cells regulate overall immune response. **(M-S)**

▶ Serum levels of aspartate aminotransferase and alanine aminotransferase reveal whether the liver is adequately detoxifying medications. **(M-S)**

▶ Serum sodium levels normally range from 135 to 145 mEq/L. **(M-S)**

▶ Serum potassium levels normally range from 3.5 to 5.0 mEq/L. **(M-S)**

▶ A patient taking prednisone (Deltasone) should consume a salt-restricted diet that is rich in potassium and protein. **(M-S)**

▶ A nurse who performs continuous ambulatory peritoneal dialysis must use sterile technique when caring for the catheter, send a peritoneal fluid sample for culture and sensitivity testing every 24 hours, and report signs of infection and fluid imbalance. **(M-S)**

▶ The Minnesota Multiphasic Personality Inventory consists of 550 statements for the subject to interpret. It assesses personality and detects disorders, such as depression and schizophrenia, in adolescents and adults. **(PSY)**

▶ TORCH infections include toxoplasmosis, other diseases (chlamydia, group B beta-hemolytic streptococcus, syphilis, and varicella zoster), rubella, cytomegalovirus, and herpesvirus. Because these infections can harm an embryo or a fetus, the nurse assesses for these in a pregnant patient or one considering pregnancy. **(MAT)**

▶ An infant infected with human immunodeficiency virus during gestation typically begins to show signs and symptoms, such as fever, adenopathy, rash, diarrhea, and failure to thrive, between ages 2 and 4 months. **(PED)**

▶ When working with patients who have acquired immunodeficiency syndrome, the nurse should wear goggles and a mask only if the possibility exists that blood or some other body fluid will splash on the nurse's face. **(M-S)**

▶ Blood spills that are infected with human immunodeficiency virus should be cleaned up with a 1:10 solution of sodium hypochlorite 5.25% (household bleach). **(M-S)**

▶ Raynaud's phenomenon is intermittent ischemic attacks in the fingers or toes marked by severe pallor and, sometimes, paresthesia and pain. **(M-S)**

▶ Intussusception (prolapse of one bowel segment into the lumen of another) causes the sudden onset of epigastric pain, sausage-shaped abdominal swelling, passage of mucus and blood through the rectum, shock, and hypotension. **(M-S)**

▶ The mechanics of delivery are engagement, descent and flexion, internal rotation, extension, external rotation, restitution, and expulsion. **(MAT)**

▶ Bence Jones protein occurs almost exclusively in the urine of patients with multiple myeloma. **(M-S)**

▶ Gaucher's disease is an autosomal disorder characterized by abnormal accumulation of glucocerebrosides (lipid substances that contain a glucose sugar) in monocytes and macrocytes. It occurs in three forms: type 1 is the adult form; type 2, the infantile form; and type 3, the juvenile form. **(M-S)**

▶ A patient with colon obstruction may develop lower abdominal pain, constipation, increasing distention, and vomiting. **(M-S)**

▶ Cold packs are applied for the first 20 to 48 hours after an injury; then heat is applied. During cold application, the pack is applied for 20 minutes and then removed for 10 to 15 minutes to prevent reflex dilation (rebound phenomenon) and frostbite injury. **(FND)**

► Colchicine (Colsalide) relieves inflammation and is used to treat gout. **(M-S)**

► Some people develop gout secondary to hyperuricemia because they can't metabolize and excrete purines normally. **(M-S)**

► A normal sperm count ranges from 20 to 150 million/ml. **(M-S)**

► Organic brain syndrome is the most common form of mental illness in elderly patients. **(PSY)**

► Clues to physical abuse of a child include inconsistent stories from parents about how the injuries occurred, lack of permission for the child to speak, wounds that don't match the stated cause of injury or multiple wounds at various stages of healing, and unexplained injuries. **(PED)**

► A first-degree burn involves the stratum corneum layer of the epidermis and is manifested as pain and redness. **(M-S)**

► Sheehan's syndrome is hypopituitarism caused by a pituitary infarct after postpartum shock and hemorrhage. **(M-S)**

► When caring for a patient with an asthma attack, the nurse should place the patient in Fowler's or semi-Fowler's position. **(M-S)**

► Among elderly patients, the incidence of noncompliance with prescribed drug therapy is high because many elderly patients have diminished visual acuity, hearing loss, or forgetfulness or need to take multiple drugs. **(M-S)**

► Tuberculosis is a reportable communicable disease caused by infection with *Mycobacterium tuberculosis* (an acid-fast bacillus). **(M-S)**

► For right-sided cardiac catheterization, the doctor passes a multilumen catheter through the superior or inferior vena cava. **(M-S)**

▶ A probable sign of pregnancy, McDonald's sign is characterized by an ease in flexing the body of the uterus against the cervix. **(MAT)**

▶ Amenorrhea is a probable sign of pregnancy. **(MAT)**

▶ A pregnant woman's partner should avoid introducing air into the vagina during oral sex because of the possibility of air embolism. **(MAT)**

▶ The presence of human chorionic gonadotropin in the blood or urine is a probable sign of pregnancy. **(MAT)**

▶ Radiography usually isn't used in a pregnant patient because it may harm the developing fetus. However, if radiography is essential, it should be performed only after 36 weeks' gestation. **(MAT)**

▶ After a fracture, bone healing occurs in these stages: hematoma formation, cellular proliferation and callus formation, and ossification and remodeling. **(M-S)**

▶ A pregnant patient who has experienced membrane rupture or vaginal bleeding shouldn't engage in sexual intercourse. **(MAT)**

▶ A patient scheduled for positron emission tomography should avoid alcohol, tobacco, and caffeine for 24 hours before the test. **(M-S)**

▶ Milia may occur as pinpoint spots over a neonate's nose. **(MAT)**

▶ In a cerebrovascular accident, decreased oxygen destroys brain cells. **(M-S)**

▶ The duration of a contraction is timed from the moment the uterine muscle begins to tense to the moment it reaches full relaxation and is measured in seconds. **(MAT)**

▶ A person with an IQ of less than 20 is profoundly retarded and considered a total-care patient. **(PSY)**

▶ The union of a male and a female gamete produces a zygote, which divides into the fertilized ovum. **(MAT)**

▶ A patient with glaucoma shouldn't receive atropine sulfate because this drug increases intraocular pressure.   **(M-S)**

▶ The nurse should instruct a hyperventilating patient to rebreathe into a paper bag.   **(M-S)**

▶ The first menstrual flow is called menarche and may be anovulatory (infertile).   **(M-S)**

▶ The pons is located above the medulla and consists of white matter (sensory and motor tracts) and gray matter (reflex centers).   **(FND)**

▶ During intermittent positive-pressure breathing, the patient should bite down on the mouthpiece, breathe normally, and let the machine do the work. After inspiration, the patient should hold his breath for 3 or 4 seconds and exhale completely through the mouthpiece.   **(M-S)**

▶ The autonomic nervous system controls the smooth muscles.   **(FND)**

▶ A patient who sits in a wheelchair for a long time may develop flexion contractures of the hips.   **(M-S)**

▶ Nystagmus is rapid horizontal or rotating eye movement. **(M-S)**

▶ After myelography, a patient should remain recumbent for 24 hours.   **(M-S)**

▶ The treatment for sprains and strains consists of immediately applying ice and elevating the arm or leg above heart level.   **(M-S)**

▶ An anticholinesterase agent shouldn't be prescribed for a patient taking morphine because it can potentiate the effect of morphine and cause respiratory depression.   **(M-S)**

▶ The primary purpose of play therapy for a hospitalized child is to allow the expression of feelings and frustrations.   **(PED)**

▶ Reframing is a therapeutic technique used with depressed patients to help them to view a situation in alternative ways. **(PSY)**

▶ A correctly written patient goal expresses the desired patient behavior, criteria for measurement, time frame for achievement, and conditions under which the behavior will occur. It is developed in collaboration with the patient. **(FND)**

▶ Percussion produces five basic notes: tympany (loud intensity, as heard over a gastric air bubble or puffed out cheek), hyperresonance (very loud, as heard over an emphysematous lung), resonance (loud, as heard over a normal lung), dullness (medium intensity, as heard over the liver or other solid organ), and flatness (soft, as heard over the thigh). **(FND)**

▶ Myopia is nearsightedness; hyperopia and presbyopia are two types of farsightedness. **(M-S)**

▶ The optic disk is yellowish pink and circular with a distinct border. **(FND)**

▶ The most effective contraceptive method is one that the woman selects for herself and uses consistently. **(M-S)**

▶ Weber's test evaluates bone conduction by placing a vibrating tuning fork on top of the patient's head at midline. The patient should perceive the sound equally in both ears. If the patient has conductive hearing loss, the sound will be heard in (lateralizes to) the ear that has conductive loss. **(M-S)**

▶ The Rinne test evaluates bone conduction by placing a vibrating tuning fork on the mastoid process of the temporal bone and air conduction by holding the vibrating tuning fork ½″ (1.3 cm) from the external auditory meatus until it is no longer heard. **(M-S)**

▶ A primary disability results from a pathologic process; a secondary disability, from inactivity. **(FND)**

▶ After an amputation, the stump may shrink because of muscle atrophy and decreased subcutaneous fat. **(M-S)**

▶ For a patient with deep vein thrombosis, heparin is used for 7 to 10 days, followed by 12 weeks of warfarin (Coumadin). **(M-S)**

► After pneumonectomy, the patient should be positioned on the operative side or on the back with the head slightly elevated. **(M-S)**

► To reduce the possibility of new emboli formation or expansion, a patient with deep vein thrombosis should receive heparin. **(M-S)**

► Atherosclerosis is the most common cause of coronary artery disease and usually involves the aorta and the femoral, coronary, and cerebral arteries. **(M-S)**

► Pulmonary embolism is a potentially fatal complication of deep vein thrombosis. **(M-S)**

► Chest pain is the most common symptom of pulmonary embolism. **(M-S)**

► The nurse should inform a patient taking phenazopyridine hydrochloride (Pyridium) that this medication colors urine orange or red. **(M-S)**

► Pneumothorax is a serious complication of central venous line placement; it is caused by inadvertent lung puncture. **(M-S)**

► *Pneumocystis carinii* pneumonia isn't considered contagious because it only affects patients with a suppressed immune system. **(M-S)**

► To enhance drug absorption, the patient should take regular erythromycin tablets with a full glass of water 1 hour before or 2 hours after a meal or should take enteric-coated tablets with food. The patient should avoid taking either type of tablets with fruit juice. **(M-S)**

► Trismus, a sign of tetanus (lockjaw), is manifested in painful spasms of masticatory muscles, difficulty opening the mouth, neck rigidity and stiffness, and dysphagia. **(M-S)**

► Nurses usually are held liable for failing to keep an accurate count of sponges and other devices during surgery. **(FND)**

► The best dietary sources of vitamin B_6 are liver, kidney, pork, soybeans, corn, and whole-grain cereals. **(FND)**

▶ The nurse should place the patient in an upright position for thoracentesis. If this isn't possible, the nurse should position the patient on the unaffected side. **(M-S)**

▶ The nurse should hang a blood bag 3′ (1 m) above the level of the planned venipuncture site if gravity flow is used. **(M-S)**

▶ The nurse should place a patient with a closed chest drainage in semi-Fowler's position. **(M-S)**

▶ Iron-rich foods, such as organ meats, nuts, legumes, dried fruit, leafy vegetables, eggs, and whole grains, generally have a low water content. **(FND)**

▶ If blood isn't transfused within 30 minutes, the nurse should return it to the blood bank because the refrigeration facilities on a nursing unit are inadequate for storing blood products. **(M-S)**

▶ Blood that is discolored and contains gas bubbles is contaminated with bacteria and shouldn't be transfused. Fifty percent of patients who receive contaminated blood die. **(M-S)**

▶ For massive, rapid blood transfusions and for exchange transfusions in neonates, blood should be warmed to 98.7° F (37° C). **(M-S)**

▶ A chest tube permits air and fluid drainage from the pleural space. **(M-S)**

▶ A hand-held resuscitation bag is an inflatable device that can be attached to a face mask or endotracheal or tracheostomy tube; it allows manual delivery of oxygen to the lungs of a patient who can't breathe independently. **(M-S)**

▶ Mechanical ventilation artificially controls or assists respiration. **(M-S)**

▶ The nurse should encourage a patient with a closed chest drainage system to cough frequently and breathe deeply to help drain the pleural space and expand the lungs. **(M-S)**

▶ Tracheal suction removes secretions from the trachea and bronchi by means of a suction catheter. **(M-S)**

▶ During colostomy irrigation, the irrigation bag should be hung 18″ (46 cm) above the stoma.   **(M-S)**

▶ The water used for colostomy irrigation should be 100° to 105° F (37.8° to 40.6° C).   **(M-S)**

▶ An arterial embolism may cause pain, loss of sensory nerves, pallor, coolness, paralysis, pulselessness, or paresthesia in the affected arm or leg.   **(M-S)**

▶ Respiratory alkalosis results from conditions that cause hyperventilation and reduce the carbon dioxide level in the arterial blood.   **(M-S)**

▶ Mineral oil is contraindicated in a patient with appendicitis, acute surgical abdomen, fecal impaction, or intestinal obstruction.   **(M-S)**

▶ When using a Y-type administration set to transfuse packed red blood cells (RBCs), the nurse can add normal saline solution to the bag to dilute the RBCs and make them less viscous.   **(M-S)**

▶ Autotransfusion is the collection, filtration, and reinfusion of the patient's own blood.   **(M-S)**

▶ Collaboration refers to joint communication and decision making between nurses and doctors designed to meet patients' needs by integrating the care regimens of both professions in one comprehensive approach.   **(FND)**

▶ Bradycardia refers to a heart rate of fewer than 60 beats/ minute.   **(FND)**

▶ A nursing diagnosis is a statement of a patient's actual or potential health problems that can be resolved, diminished, or otherwise changed by nursing interventions.   **(FND)**

▶ During the assessment phase of the nursing process, the nurse collects and analyzes three types of data: health history, physical examination, and laboratory and diagnostic test data.   **(FND)**

▶ The patient's health history consists primarily of subjective data—information supplied by the patient. **(FND)**

▶ The physical examination includes objective data obtained by inspection, palpation, percussion, and auscultation. **(FND)**

▶ When documenting patient care, the nurse should write legibly, use only standard abbreviations, and sign every entry. The nurse should never destroy or attempt to obliterate documentation or leave vacant lines. **(FND)**

▶ Factors that affect body temperature include time of day, age, physical activity, phase of menstrual cycle, and pregnancy. **(FND)**

▶ The most accessible and commonly used artery for measuring a patient's pulse rate is the radial artery, which is compressed against the radius to take the pulse rate. **(FND)**

▶ The normal pulse rate of a resting adult is 60 to 100 beats/minute. The rate is slightly faster in women than in men and much faster in children than in adults. **(FND)**

▶ Prepared I.V. solutions fall into three general categories: isotonic, hypotonic, and hypertonic. Isotonic solutions possess a solute concentration similar to body fluids; their addition to plasma doesn't change plasma osmolarity. Hypotonic solutions have a lower osmotic pressure than body fluids; their addition decreases plasma osmolarity. Hypertonic solutions have a higher osmotic pressure than body fluids; their addition increases plasma osmolarity. **(M-S)**

▶ Stress incontinence refers to involuntary urine leakage triggered by a sudden physical strain, such as a cough, sneeze, or quick movement. **(M-S)**

▶ Laboratory test results are an objective form of assessment data. **(FND)**

▶ Decreased renal function makes an elderly patient more susceptible to the development of renal calculi. **(M-S)**

▶ Because elderly patients experience subcutaneous tissue redistribution and loss in areas such as the buttocks and deltoid muscles, the nurse should consider using shorter needles for injection of medication. **(M-S)**

▶ Urge incontinence refers to the inability to suppress a sudden urge to urinate. **(M-S)**

▶ Total incontinence is continuous and uncontrollable urine leakage resulting from the bladder's inability to retain urine. **(M-S)**

▶ Protein, vitamin, and mineral needs usually remain constant as a person ages, but caloric requirements decrease. **(M-S)**

▶ Four valves keep blood flowing in one direction in the heart: two atrioventricular valves (tricuspid and mitral) and two semilunar valves (pulmonic and aortic). **(M-S)**

▶ An elderly patient's height may decrease because of narrowing of the intervertebral spaces and exaggerated spinal curvature. **(M-S)**

▶ The measurement systems most often used in clinical practice are the metric system, apothecaries' system, and household system. **(FND)**

▶ Before signing an informed consent, a patient should know whether other treatment options are available and should understand what will occur during the preoperative, intraoperative, and postoperative phases; the risks involved; and the possible complications. The patient also should have a general idea of the time required from surgery to recovery and should have an opportunity to ask questions. **(FND)**

▶ A patient must sign a separate informed consent form for each procedure. **(FND)**

▶ Constipation most commonly occurs when the urge to defecate is suppressed and the muscles associated with bowel movements remain contracted. **(M-S)**

▶ Gout develops in four stages: asymptomatic, acute, intercritical, and chronic. **(M-S)**

▶ During percussion, the nurse uses quick, sharp tapping of the fingers or hands against body surfaces to produce sounds (that help determine the size, shape, position, and density of underlying organs and tissues), elicit tenderness, or assess reflexes. **(FND)**

▶ Ballottement is a form of light palpation involving gentle, repetitive bouncing of tissues against the hand and feeling their rebound. **(FND)**

▶ A foot cradle keeps bed linen off the patient's feet, which prevents skin irritation and breakdown, especially in a patient with peripheral vascular disease or neuropathy. **(FND)**

▶ If the patient is a married minor, permission to perform a procedure can be obtained from the patient's spouse. **(FND)**

▶ Gastric lavage is the flushing of the stomach and removal of ingested substances through a nasogastric tube. It can be used to treat poisoning or drug overdose. **(FND)**

▶ Common postoperative complications include hemorrhage, infection, hypovolemia, septicemia, septic shock, atelectasis, pneumonia, thrombophlebitis, and pulmonary embolism. **(M-S)**

▶ An insulin pump delivers a continuous infusion of insulin into a selected subcutaneous site, commonly in the abdomen. **(M-S)**

▶ During the evaluation step of the nursing process, the nurse assesses the patient's response to therapy. **(FND)**

▶ A common symptom of salicylate (aspirin) toxicity is tinnitus (ringing in the ears). **(M-S)**

▶ A frostbitten extremity needs to be rapidly thawed even if it means delaying definitive treatments. **(M-S)**

▶ Bruits commonly indicate a life- or limb-threatening vascular disease. **(FND)**

▶ A patient with Raynaud's disease shouldn't smoke cigarettes or other tobacco products. **(M-S)**

▶ O.U. means each eye; O.D., right eye; and O.S., left eye. **(FND)**

▶ Raynaud's disease is a primary arteriospastic disorder with no known cause; Raynaud's phenomenon, however, is caused by another disorder, such as scleroderma.   **(M-S)**

▶ To remove a foreign body from the eye, the nurse should irrigate the eye with sterile normal saline solution.   **(M-S)**

▶ When irrigating the eye, the nurse should direct the solution toward the lower conjunctival sac.   **(M-S)**

▶ Emergency care for a corneal injury from a caustic substance is eye flushing with copious amounts of water for 20 to 30 minutes.   **(M-S)**

▶ To remove a patient's artificial eye, the nurse depresses the lower lid.   **(FND)**

▶ The nurse should use a warm saline solution to clean an artificial eye.   **(FND)**

▶ Debridement is the mechanical, chemical, or surgical removal of necrotic tissue from a wound.   **(M-S)**

▶ Severe pain after cataract surgery indicates bleeding in the eye.   **(M-S)**

▶ The bivalve cast is cut into anterior and posterior portions to allow skin inspection.   **(M-S)**

▶ After ear irrigation, the nurse should place the patient on the affected side to permit gravity to drain fluid that remains in the ear.   **(M-S)**

▶ In evaluating dehydration in an infant, the nurse should assess skin turgor on the inner thigh.   **(PED)**

▶ A thready pulse is very fine and scarcely perceptible.   **(FND)**

▶ If a patient with an indwelling catheter reports abdominal discomfort, the nurse should assess for bladder distention, which may be caused by catheter blockage.   **(M-S)**

▶ Continuous bladder irrigation helps prevent urinary tract obstruction by flushing out small blood clots that form after prostate or bladder surgery. **(M-S)**

▶ The nurse should remove an indwelling catheter when bladder decompression is no longer needed, when the catheter is obstructed, or when the patient can resume voiding. (The longer a catheter remains in place, the greater the risk of urinary tract infection.) **(M-S)**

▶ The extent of a burn injury in an adult can be determined by using the Rule of Nines: the head and neck are counted as 9%; each arm, as 9%; each leg, as 18%; the back of the trunk, as 18%; the front of the trunk, as 18%; and the perineum, as 1%. **(M-S)**

▶ In a deep partial-thickness burn, the epidermis and dermis are affected. **(M-S)**

▶ Axillary temperature usually is 1° F lower than oral temperature. **(FND)**

▶ After suctioning a tracheostomy tube, the nurse must document the color, amount, consistency, and odor of secretions. **(FND)**

▶ Nursing interventions for an asthma attack include administering oxygen and bronchodilators as prescribed, placing the patient in semi-Fowler's position, encouraging diaphragmatic breathing, and helping the patient relax. **(M-S)**

▶ On a medication prescription, the abbreviation p.c. means that the medication should be administered after meals. **(FND)**

▶ After bladder irrigation, the nurse should document the amount, color, and clarity of the urine and the presence of clots or sediment. **(FND)**

▶ Prostate cancer usually is fatal if bone metastasis occurs. **(M-S)**

▶ Laws regarding patient self-determination vary from state to state. Therefore, the nurse must be familiar with the laws of the state in which she works. **(FND)**

▶ Gauge refers to the inside diameter of a needle. The smaller the gauge, the larger the diameter.   **(FND)**

▶ An adult normally has 32 permanent teeth.   **(FND)**

▶ After turning a patient, the nurse should document the position used, time turned, and skin assessment findings.   **(FND)**

▶ A strict vegetarian needs vitamin B_{12} supplements because animals and animal products are the only source of this vitamin.   **(M-S)**

▶ PERRLA is an abbreviation for normal pupil assessment findings: pupils equal, round, and reactive to light with accommodation.   **(FND)**

▶ When percussing a patient's chest for postural drainage, the nurse's hands should be cupped.   **(FND)**

▶ Regular insulin is the only insulin that can be mixed with other types of insulins and can be given intravenously.   **(M-S)**

▶ If a patient pulls out the outer tracheostomy tube, the nurse should hold open the tracheostomy with a surgical dilator until the doctor provides appropriate care.   **(M-S)**

▶ When measuring a patient's pulse, the nurse should assess the rate, rhythm, quality, and strength.   **(FND)**

▶ Before transferring a patient from a bed to a wheelchair, the nurse should push the wheelchair's footrests to the sides and lock its wheels.   **(FND)**

▶ Tetralogy of Fallot consists of four defects: ventricular septal defect, overriding aorta, pulmonic stenosis, and right ventricular hypertrophy.   **(PED)**

▶ When assessing respirations, the nurse should document the rate, rhythm, depth, and quality.   **(FND)**

▶ For a subcutaneous injection, the nurse should use a ⅝" 25G needle.   **(FND)**

▶ The medulla oblongata is the part of the brain that controls the respiratory center. **(M-S)**

▶ For an unconscious patient, the nurse should perform passive range-of-motion exercises every 2 to 4 hours. **(M-S)**

▶ Timed-release medication isn't recommended for use with a patient who has an ileostomy because it releases the drug at different rates along the GI tract. **(M-S)**

▶ The notation "AA & O × 3" indicates that the patient is awake, alert, and oriented to person (knows who he is), place (knows where he is), and time (knows the date and time). **(FND)**

▶ Fluid intake includes all fluids taken by mouth, including foods that are liquid at room temperature, such as gelatin, custard, and ice cream; I.V. fluids; and fluids administered in feeding tubes. Fluid output includes urine, vomitus, and drainage (such as from a nasogastric tube or from a wound) as well as blood loss, diarrhea or stool, and perspiration. **(FND)**

▶ The nurse isn't required to wear gloves when applying nitroglycerin paste; however, the nurse should wash her hands after applying the medication. **(M-S)**

▶ A patient's fluid intake usually is restricted after midnight before intravenous pyelography. **(M-S)**

▶ After administering an intradermal injection, the nurse shouldn't massage the area because massage can irritate the site and interfere with results. **(FND)**

▶ When administering an intradermal injection, the nurse should hold the syringe almost flat against the patient's skin (at about a 15-degree angle) with the bevel up. **(FND)**

▶ After a thyroidectomy, the patient should remain in semi-Fowler's position with the head firmly supported by pillows; neck flexion should be avoided. **(M-S)**

▶ To obtain an accurate blood pressure, the nurse should inflate the manometer 20 to 30 mm Hg above the disappearance of the radial pulse before releasing the cuff pressure. **(FND)**

▶ A sodium polystyrene sulfonate (Kayexalate) enema, which exchanges sodium ions for potassium ions, is used to decrease the potassium level in a patient with hyperkalemia. **(M-S)**

▶ If the color of a stoma is much lighter than when previously assessed, decreased circulation to the stoma should be suspected. **(M-S)**

▶ Massage is contraindicated in a leg with a blood clot because it may dislodge the clot. **(M-S)**

▶ The first place a nurse can detect jaundice in an adult is in the sclera of the eye. **(M-S)**

▶ Jaundice is caused by excessive levels of conjugated or unconjugated bilirubin in the blood. **(M-S)**

▶ Mydriatic drugs are used primarily to dilate the pupils for intraocular examinations. **(M-S)**

▶ After eye surgery, the patient should be placed on the unaffected side. **(M-S)**

▶ When assigning tasks to a licensed practical nurse, the registered nurse should delegate tasks that are considered bedside nursing care, such as taking vital signs, changing simple dressings, and giving baths. **(M-S)**

▶ Deep calf pain on dorsiflexion of the foot is a positive Homans' sign, which suggests venous thrombosis or thrombophlebitis. **(M-S)**

▶ Ultra short-acting barbiturates, such as thiopental sodium (Pentothal), are used as injection anesthetics in situations that require a short duration of anesthesia such as outpatient surgery. **(M-S)**

▶ Atropine sulfate may be used as a preanesthesia medication to reduce secretions and minimize vagal reflexes. **(M-S)**

▶ The nursing care plan for a patient with infectious mononucleosis should emphasize strict bed rest during the acute febrile stage to ensure adequate rest. **(M-S)**

▶ During the acute phase of infectious mononucleosis, the patient should curtail activities to minimize the possibility of rupturing the enlarged spleen. **(M-S)**

▶ Daily application of a long-acting, transdermal nitroglycerin patch is a convenient, effective way to prevent chronic angina. **(M-S)**

▶ Fluoxetine (Prozac), sertraline (Zoloft), and paroxetine (Paxil) are serotonin reuptake inhibitors used in the treatment of depression. **(PSY)**

▶ The nurse must wear a cap, gloves, gown, and mask when providing wound care to a patient with third-degree burns. **(M-S)**

▶ The nurse should expect to administer an analgesic before bathing a burn patient. **(M-S)**

▶ The passage of black, tarry stools (melena) is a common sign of lower GI bleeding but also may occur in upper GI bleeding. **(M-S)**

▶ The nurse should count an irregular pulse for 1 full minute. **(FND)**

▶ Spermatozoa (or their fragments) remain in the vagina for 72 hours after sexual intercourse. **(MAT)**

▶ A patient with a gastric ulcer should avoid aspirin and aspirin-containing products because they can irritate the gastric mucosa. **(M-S)**

▶ A patient who is vomiting while lying down should be placed in a lateral position to prevent aspiration of vomitus. **(FND)**

▶ While administering chemotherapy agents by an I.V. line, the nurse should discontinue the infusion at the first sign of extravasation. **(M-S)**

▶ A low-fiber diet may contribute to the development of hemorrhoids. **(M-S)**

▶ A patient with abdominal pain shouldn't receive an analgesic until the cause of the pain is determined. **(M-S)**

▶ If surgery requires hair removal, the Centers for Disease Control and Prevention recommends that a depilatory be used to avoid skin abrasions and cuts. **(M-S)**

▶ For nasotracheal suctioning, the nurse should set wall suction at 50 to 95 mm Hg for an infant, 95 to 115 mm Hg for a child, or 80 to 120 mm Hg for an adult. **(M-S)**

▶ The hallmark of tetralogy of Fallot is cyanosis, which usually appears several months after birth but may be present at birth if the infant has severe pulmonary stenosis. **(PED)**

▶ A change in pulse rate and rhythm may signal the onset of fatal arrhythmias in a patient who has had a myocardial infarction. **(M-S)**

▶ Treatment for epistaxis includes nasal packing, ice packs, cautery with silver nitrate, and pressure on the nares. **(M-S)**

▶ Prophylaxis is disease prevention. **(FND)**

▶ Palliative treatment relieves or reduces the intensity of uncomfortable symptoms but doesn't cure the causative disorder. **(M-S)**

▶ Placing a postoperative patient in an upright position too quickly may produce hypotension. **(M-S)**

▶ Body alignment is achieved when the body parts are in proper relation to their natural position. **(FND)**

▶ Verapamil (Calan) and diltiazem (Cardizem) slow the inflow of calcium to the heart, thereby decreasing the risk of supraventricular tachycardia. **(M-S)**

▶ Trust is the foundation of a nurse-patient relationship. **(FND)**

▶ Blood pressure is the force exerted by the circulating volume of blood on arterial walls. **(FND)**

▶ Patient outcomes following cardiopulmonary bypass graft include turning, coughing, deep breathing, use of assistive breathing devices, and wound splinting. **(M-S)**

▶ A patient exposed to hepatitis B should receive 0.06 ml/kg I.M. of immune globulin within 72 hours after exposure and a repeat dose at 28 days after exposure. **(M-S)**

▶ The nurse should advise a patient undergoing radiation therapy not to remove the markings on the skin made by the radiation therapist because these markings are landmarks for treatment. **(M-S)**

▶ The most common symptom of osteoarthritis is joint pain—particularly after exercise or weight bearing—that usually is relieved by rest. **(M-S)**

▶ Malpractice refers to a professional's wrongful conduct, improper discharge of duties, or failure to meet standards of care, which causes harm to another. **(FND)**

▶ In adults, urine volume normally ranges from 800 to 2,000 ml/day and averages between 1,200 and 1,500 ml/day. **(M-S)**

▶ As a general rule, nurses can't refuse a patient care assignment; however, they may refuse to participate in abortions in most states. **(FND)**

▶ A nurse can be found negligent if a patient is injured because the nurse failed to perform a duty that a reasonable and prudent person would perform or because the nurse performed an act that a reasonable and prudent person wouldn't perform. **(FND)**

▶ Directly applied moist heat softens crusts and exudates, penetrates deeper than dry heat, doesn't dry the skin, and usually is more comfortable for the patient. **(M-S)**

▶ Tetracyclines seldom are considered drugs of choice for most common bacterial infections because their overuse has led to the emergence of tetracycline-resistant bacteria. **(M-S)**

▶ Because light degrades nitroprusside (Nitropress), the drug must be shielded from light. For example, an I.V. bag containing nitroprusside sodium should be wrapped in foil. **(M-S)**

▶ Cephalosporins should be used cautiously in patients who are allergic to penicillin because such patients are more susceptible to hypersensitivity reactions. **(M-S)**

▶ If chloramphenicol and penicillin must be administered concomitantly, the nurse should give the penicillin 1 or more hours before the chloramphenicol to avoid reduction in penicillin's bactericidal activity. **(M-S)**

▶ The erythrocyte sedimentation rate measures the distance and speed that erythrocytes in whole blood have fallen in a vertical tube in 1 hour. The rate at which they fall to the bottom of the tube corresponds to the degree of inflammation. **(M-S)**

▶ When teaching a patient with myasthenia gravis about pyridostigmine bromide (Mestinon) therapy, the nurse should stress the importance of taking the medication exactly as prescribed, on time, and in evenly spaced doses to prevent a relapse and maximize the effect of the drug. **(M-S)**

▶ If an antibiotic must be administered into a peripheral heparin lock, the nurse should flush the site with normal saline solution after the infusion to maintain I.V. patency. **(M-S)**

▶ The nurse should instruct a patient with angina to take a nitroglycerin tablet before anticipated stress or exercise or, if the angina is nocturnal, at bedtime. **(M-S)**

▶ Arterial blood gas analysis evaluates gas exchange in the lungs (alveolar ventilation) by measuring the partial pressures of oxygen and carbon dioxide and the pH of an arterial sample. **(M-S)**

▶ The normal serum magnesium level ranges from 1.7 to 2.1 mg/dl or 1.5 to 2.5 mEq/L. **(M-S)**

▶ Patient preparation for a total cholesterol test includes an overnight fast and abstinence from alcohol for 24 hours before the test. **(M-S)**

▶ The fasting plasma glucose test measures glucose levels after a 12- to 14-hour fast. **(M-S)**

▶ The normal blood pH ranges from 7.35 to 7.45. A blood pH higher than 7.45 indicates alkalemia; one lower than 7.35 indicates acidemia. **(M-S)**

▶ During the acid perfusion test, a small amount of weak hydrochloric acid solution is infused by way of a nasoesophageal tube. A positive test result (pain after infusion) suggests reflux esophagitis. **(M-S)**

▶ Normally, the partial pressure of arterial carbon dioxide ($Paco_2$) ranges from 35 to 45 mm Hg. A $Paco_2$ greater than 45 mm Hg indicates acidemia secondary to hypoventilation; one less than 35 mm Hg indicates alkalemia secondary to hyperventilation. **(M-S)**

▶ Red cell indices aid in the diagnosis and classification of anemias. **(M-S)**

▶ Normally, the partial pressure of arterial oxygen (Pao_2) ranges from 80 to 100 mm Hg. A Pao_2 between 50 and 80 mm Hg indicates respiratory insufficiency. Pao_2 less than 50 mm Hg indicates respiratory failure. **(M-S)**

▶ The white blood cell (WBC) differential evaluates WBC distribution and morphology and provides more specific information about a patient's immune system than the WBC count. **(M-S)**

▶ An exercise stress test (treadmill test, exercise electrocardiogram) continues until the patient reaches a predetermined target heart rate or experiences chest pain, fatigue, or other signs of exercise intolerance. **(M-S)**

▶ Alterable risk factors for coronary artery disease include cigarette smoking, hypertension, high cholesterol or triglyceride levels, and diabetes. **(M-S)**

▶ The mediastinum is the space between the lungs that contains the heart, esophagus, trachea, and other structures. **(M-S)**

▶ Major complications of acute myocardial infarction include arrhythmias, acute heart failure, cardiogenic shock, thromboembolism, and left ventricular rupture. **(M-S)**

► The sinoatrial node is a cluster of hundreds of cells located in the right atrial wall near the opening of the superior vena cava. **(M-S)**

► For one-person cardiopulmonary resuscitation, the ratio of compressions to ventilations is 15:2. **(M-S)**

► For two-person cardiopulmonary resuscitation, the ratio of compressions to ventilations is 5:1. **(M-S)**

► A patient with pulseless ventricular tachycardia is a candidate for cardioversion. **(M-S)**

► Echocardiography, a noninvasive test that directs ultra-high-frequency sound waves through the chest wall into the heart, evaluates cardiac structure and function and can reveal valve deformities, tumors, septal defects, pericardial effusion, and hypertrophic cardiomyopathy. **(M-S)**

► Ataxia refers to an impaired ability to coordinate movements and results from a cerebellar or spinal cord lesion. **(M-S)**

► On an electrocardiogram strip, each small block on the horizontal axis represents 0.04 second. Each large block (composed of five small blocks) represents 0.2 second. **(M-S)**

► Starling's law states that the force of contraction of each heartbeat depends on the length of the muscle fibers of the heart wall. **(M-S)**

► The therapeutic blood level for digoxin is 0.5 to 2.5 ng/ml. **(M-S)**

► Pancrelipase (Pancrease) is used to treat cystic fibrosis and chronic pancreatitis. **(M-S)**

► Treatment for mild to moderate varicose veins includes antiembolism stockings and an exercise program with walking to minimize venous pooling. **(M-S)**

► According to Erikson, a young adult (ages 19 to 35) is in the developmental stage of intimacy versus isolation. **(PED)**

▶ States have enacted good Samaritan laws to encourage professionals to provide medical assistance at the scene of an accident without fear of a lawsuit arising from such assistance. These laws don't apply to care provided in a health care facility. **(FND)**

▶ A doctor should sign verbal and telephone orders within the time established by institutional policy, usually within 24 hours. **(FND)**

▶ A competent adult has the right to refuse lifesaving medical treatment; however, the individual should be fully informed of the consequences of this refusal. **(FND)**

▶ An intoxicated patient isn't considered competent for the purposes of refusing required medical treatment and shouldn't be allowed to check out of a hospital against medical advice. **(M-S)**

▶ The primary difference between the pain of angina and a myocardial infarction is the duration of pain. **(M-S)**

▶ Although a patient's health record or chart is the health care facility's physical property, its contents belong to the patient. **(FND)**

▶ Before a patient's record can be released to a third party, the patient or the patient's legal guardian must give written consent. **(FND)**

▶ Under the Controlled Substances Act, every dose of a controlled drug dispensed by the pharmacy must be accounted for, whether the dose was administered to a particular patient or discarded accidentally. **(FND)**

▶ A nurse can't perform duties that violate a rule or regulation established by a state licensing board even if it is authorized by a health care facility or doctor. **(FND)**

▶ The nurse should select a private room, preferably with a door that can be closed, to minimize interruptions during a patient interview. **(FND)**

▶ In categorizing nursing diagnoses, the nurse should address actual life-threatening problems first, followed by potentially life-threatening concerns. **(FND)**

▶ The major components of a nursing care plan are outcome criteria (patient goals) and nursing interventions. **(FND)**

▶ Standing orders, or protocols, establish guidelines for treating a particular disease or set of symptoms. **(FND)**

▶ Prolactin stimulates and sustains milk production. **(MAT)**

▶ Gynecomastia refers to excessive mammary gland development and increased breast size in boys and men. **(M-S)**

▶ The early stage of Alzheimer's disease lasts from 2 to 4 years and is manifested in inappropriate affect, transient paranoia, disorientation to time, memory loss, careless dressing, and impaired judgment. **(PSY)**

▶ The middle stage of Alzheimer's disease lasts from 4 to 7 years and is marked by profound personality changes, loss of independence, disorientation, confusion, inability to recognize family members, and nocturnal restlessness. **(PSY)**

▶ The last stage of Alzheimer's disease occurs during the final year of life and is manifested in a blank facial expression, seizures, loss of appetite, emaciation, irritability, and total dependence. **(PSY)**

▶ Classic symptoms of Graves' disease are an enlarged thyroid, nervousness, heat intolerance, weight loss despite increased appetite, sweating, diarrhea, tremor, and palpitations. **(M-S)**

▶ Generalized malaise is a common symptom of viral and bacterial infections and depressive disorders. **(M-S)**

▶ Vitamin C and protein are the most important nutrients for wound healing. **(M-S)**

▶ A patient with portal hypertension should receive vitamin K to promote active thrombin formation by the liver, which reduces the risk of bleeding. **(M-S)**

▶ The nurse should administer a sedative cautiously to a patient with cirrhosis because the damaged liver can't metabolize drugs effectively.   **(M-S)**

▶ Beta-hemolytic streptococcal infections should be treated aggressively to prevent glomerulonephritis, rheumatic fever, and other complications.   **(M-S)**

▶ The most common nosocomial infection is urinary tract infection.   **(M-S)**

▶ The nurse should implement strict isolation precautions to protect a patient with a third-degree burn infected by *Staphylococcus aureus*.   **(M-S)**

▶ A patient undergoing external radiation therapy shouldn't apply cream or lotion to the treatment site.   **(M-S)**

▶ Strabismus is a normal finding in a neonate.   **(MAT)**

▶ The most common vascular complication of diabetes mellitus is atherosclerosis.   **(M-S)**

▶ Insulin deficiency may result in hyperglycemia.   **(M-S)**

▶ Signs of Parkinson's disease include drooling, masklike expression, and propulsive gait.   **(M-S)**

▶ I.V. cholangiography is contraindicated in a patient with hyperthyroidism, severe renal or hepatic damage, tuberculosis, or iodine hypersensitivity.   **(M-S)**

▶ In assessing a patient's heart, the nurse normally finds the point of maximal impulse at the fifth intercostal space near the apex.   **(FND)**

▶ The S_1 sound heard on auscultation is caused by closure of the mitral and tricuspid valves.   **(FND)**

▶ Threatening a patient with an injection for failing to take an oral medication is an example of assault.   **(PSY)**

▶ Mirrors should be removed from the room of a patient with disfiguring wounds such as those sustained with facial burns. **(M-S)**

▶ A patient with gouty arthritis should increase the fluid intake to prevent calculi formation. **(M-S)**

▶ Anxiety is the most common cause of chest pain. **(M-S)**

▶ A patient on a low-salt diet should avoid canned vegetables. **(M-S)**

▶ Bananas are a good source of potassium and should be included in a low-salt diet for a patient taking a loop diuretic such as furosemide (Lasix). **(M-S)**

▶ The nurse should encourage a patient at risk for pneumonia to turn frequently, cough, and breathe deeply. These actions mobilize pulmonary secretions, promote alveolar gas exchange, and help prevent atelectasis. **(M-S)**

▶ The nurse should notify the doctor anytime a patient's blood pressure reaches 180/100 mm Hg. **(M-S)**

▶ Buck's traction is used to immobilize and reduce spasms in a fractured hip. **(M-S)**

▶ For a patient with a fractured hip, the nurse should assess neurocirculatory status every 2 hours. **(M-S)**

▶ When caring for a patient with a fractured hip, the nurse should use pillows or trochanter roll to maintain abduction. **(M-S)**

▶ Orthopnea is a symptom of left ventricular failure. **(M-S)**

▶ Although a fiberglass cast is more durable and dries faster than a plaster cast, it frequently causes skin irritation. **(M-S)**

▶ The major circulatory complication of an immobilized patient is pulmonary embolism. **(M-S)**

▶ To relieve edema in a fractured limb, the patient should keep the limb elevated. **(M-S)**

▶ I.V. antibiotics are the treatment of choice for a patient with osteomyelitis. **(M-S)**

▶ A postpartum patient may resume sexual intercourse when perineal and uterine wounds have healed (usually within 4 weeks after delivery). **(MAT)**

▶ Blue dye in cimetidine (Tagamet) can cause a false-positive result on a fecal occult blood test such as a Hemoccult test. **(M-S)**

▶ A pregnant staff member shouldn't be assigned to work with a patient who has a cytomegalovirus infection. **(MAT)**

▶ The nurse should suspect elder abuse if wounds are inconsistent with the history, multiple wounds are present, or wounds are in different stages of healing. **(M-S)**

▶ Fetal demise refers to death of the fetus after viability. **(MAT)**

▶ Immediately after amputation, patient care includes monitoring drainage from the stump, positioning the affected arm or leg, assisting with exercises prescribed by a physical therapist, and wrapping and conditioning the stump. **(M-S)**

▶ Premature infants develop respiratory distress syndrome because their alveoli lack surfactant. **(MAT)**

▶ A patient who is prone to constipation should increase the bulk intake by eating whole-grain cereals and fresh fruits and vegetables. **(M-S)**

▶ The most common method of inducing labor after artificial rupture of the membrane is oxytocin (Pitocin) infusion. **(MAT)**

▶ The speculum used in the pelvic examination of a rape victim should be lubricated with water because commercial lubricants retard sperm motility and interfere with specimen collection and analysis. **(M-S)**

▶ Physical comfort is the top priority in nursing care for a terminally ill patient. **(M-S)**

▶ Dorsiflexion of the foot provides immediate relief of leg cramps. **(M-S)**

▶ After cardiac surgery, the patient should limit daily sodium intake to 2 g and daily cholesterol intake to 300 mg. **(M-S)**

▶ After the patient's amniotic membranes rupture, the initial nursing action is to assess the fetal heart rate. **(MAT)**

▶ Bleeding after intercourse is an early sign of cervical cancer. **(M-S)**

▶ Oral antidiabetic agents, such as chlorpropamide (Diabinese) and tolbutamide (Orinase), stimulate insulin release from beta cells in the islets of Langerhans of the pancreas. **(M-S)**

▶ When visiting a patient with a radiation implant, family members and friends must limit their stay to 10 minutes. Pregnant visitors and nurses are restricted from entering the room. **(M-S)**

▶ Common causes of vaginal infection include using an antibiotic, an oral contraceptive, or a corticosteroid; wearing tight-fitting panty hose; and having sexual intercourse with an infected partner. **(M-S)**

▶ A patient with a radiation implant should be maintained in isolation until the implant is removed. The nurse should carefully plan the time spent with the patient to minimize radiation exposure, which increases with time. **(M-S)**

▶ Among cultural groups, Native Americans have the lowest incidence of cancer. **(M-S)**

▶ The kidneys filter blood, selectively reabsorb substances needed to maintain the constancy of body fluid, and excrete metabolic wastes. **(M-S)**

▶ Reexamination of life goals is a major developmental task during middle adulthood. **(PSY)**

▶ To prevent straining during defecation, docusate sodium (Colace) is the laxative of choice for patients recovering from a myocardial infarction, rectal or cardiac surgery, or postpartum constipation. **(M-S)**

▶ Acute alcohol withdrawal is manifested by anorexia, insomnia, headache, and restlessness and escalates to a syndrome that is characterized by agitation, disorientation, vivid hallucinations, and tremors of the hands, feet, legs, and tongue. **(PSY)**

▶ In a hospitalized alcoholic, alcohol withdrawal delirium most commonly occurs 3 to 4 days after admission. **(PSY)**

▶ Confrontation is a communication technique in which the nurse points out discrepancies between the patient's words and nonverbal behaviors. **(PSY)**

▶ Telangiectatic nevi (stork bites) are normal neonatal skin lesions characterized by flat red or purple areas on the back of the neck, upper eyelids, upper lip, and bridge of the nose. They regress by age 2. **(PED)**

▶ After prostate surgery, a patient's primary sources of pain are bladder spasms and irritation in the area around the catheter. **(M-S)**

▶ Toxoplasmosis is more likely to affect a pregnant cat owner than other pregnant women because cat feces in the litter box harbor the infecting organism. **(M-S)**

▶ The most common reasons for cesarean birth are malpresentation, fetal distress, cephalopelvic disproportion, pregnancy-induced hypertension, previous cesarean birth, and inadequate progress in labor. **(MAT)**

▶ Amniocentesis increases the risk of spontaneous abortion, trauma to the fetus or placenta, premature labor, infection, and Rh sensitization of the fetus. **(MAT)**

▶ After amniocentesis, abdominal cramping or spontaneous vaginal bleeding may indicate complications. **(MAT)**

▶ An Rh-negative primagravida should receive $Rh_o(D)$ immune globulin (RhoGAM) after delivering an Rh-positive infant to prevent her from developing Rh antibodies. **(MAT)**

▶ If a pregnant patient's test results are negative for glucose but positive for acetone, the nurse should assess the patient's diet for inadequate caloric intake. **(MAT)**

▶ Calcium deficiency and lack of proper exercise can result in leg cramps during pregnancy. **(MAT)**

▶ Good food sources of folic acid include green leafy vegetables, liver, and legumes. **(M-S)**

▶ Rubella infection in a pregnant patient, especially during the first trimester, can lead to spontaneous abortion or stillbirth as well as fetal cardiac and other birth defects. **(MAT)**

▶ The Glasgow Coma Scale evaluates verbal, eye, and motor responses to determine level of consciousness. **(M-S)**

▶ The nurse should place an unconscious patient in low Fowler's position for intermittent nasogastric tube feedings. **(M-S)**

▶ Laënnec's (alcoholic) cirrhosis is the most common type of cirrhosis. **(M-S)**

▶ In decorticate posturing, the patient's arms are adducted and flexed, with the wrists and fingers flexed on the chest. The legs are stiffly extended and internally rotated, with plantar flexion of the feet. **(M-S)**

▶ For a patient with substance-induced delirium, the time of drug ingestion can help determine if the drug can be evacuated from the body. **(PSY)**

▶ A pregnant patient may receive a prescription for an iron supplement to help prevent anemia. **(MAT)**

▶ Direct antiglobulin (direct Coombs') test is used to detect maternal antibodies attached to red blood cells in the neonate. **(MAT)**

▶ The most common intra-abdominal tumor in children is Wilms' tumor (nephroblastoma). **(PED)**

▶ A patient who is a potential candidate for surgery should receive nothing by mouth from midnight of the day before surgery unless cleared by a doctor. **(M-S)**

▶ Nausea and vomiting during the first trimester of pregnancy are caused by rising levels of the hormone human chorionic gonadotropin (hCG). **(MAT)**

▶ In an infant, feeding problems, such as fatigue, tachypnea, and irritability during feeding, may be early signs of a congenital heart defect. **(PED)**

▶ Meperidine (Demerol) is an effective analgesic for relieving the pain of nephrolithiasis (urinary calculi). **(M-S)**

▶ An injured patient with thrombocytopenia is at risk for life-threatening internal and external hemorrhage. **(M-S)**

▶ The Trendelenburg test is used to check for unilateral hip dislocation. **(M-S)**

▶ As soon as possible after death, the patient should be placed in the supine position with the arms at the sides and the head on a pillow. **(M-S)**

▶ Vascular resistance depends on blood viscosity, vessel length and, most important, inside vessel diameter. **(M-S)**

▶ A below-the-knee amputation leaves the knee intact for prosthesis application and allows a more normal gait. **(M-S)**

▶ Cerebrospinal fluid flows through and protects the four ventricles of the brain, the subarachnoid space, and the spinal canal. **(M-S)**

▶ Sodium regulates extracellular osmolality. **(M-S)**

▶ The heart and brain can maintain blood circulation in the early stages of shock. **(M-S)**

▶ After limb amputation, narcotic analgesics may not relieve "phantom limb" pain. **(M-S)**

▶ A patient who receives multiple blood transfusions is at risk for developing hypocalcemia. **(M-S)**

▶ Syphilis initially causes painless chancres (small, fluid-filled lesions) on the genitals and sometimes on other parts of the body.   **(M-S)**

▶ Exposure to a radioactive source is controlled by time (limiting time spent with patient), distance (from the patient), and shield (lead apron).   **(M-S)**

▶ Jaundice is a sign of dysfunction, not a disease.   **(M-S)**

▶ Severe jaundice can result in brain stem dysfunction if the unconjugated bilirubin level in blood is elevated to 20 to 25 mg/dl.   **(M-S)**

▶ The patient should take cimetidine (Tagamet) with meals to help ensure a consistent therapeutic effect.   **(M-S)**

▶ When caring for a patient with jaundice, the nurse should relieve pruritus by providing a soothing lotion or baking soda bath and should prevent injury by keeping the patient's fingernails short.   **(M-S)**

▶ Type B hepatitis, which is generally transmitted parenterally, also can be spread through contact with human secretions and feces.   **(M-S)**

▶ Insulin is a naturally occurring hormone secreted by the beta cells of the islets of Langerhans in the pancreas in response to a rise in the blood glucose level.   **(M-S)**

▶ Diabetes mellitus is a chronic endocrine disorder characterized by insulin deficiency or resistance to insulin by body tissues.   **(M-S)**

▶ A diagnosis of diabetes mellitus is based on the classic symptoms (polyuria, polyphagia, weight loss, and polydipsia) and a random blood glucose level above 200 mg/dl or a fasting plasma glucose level above 140 mg/dl on two testings.   **(M-S)**

▶ A patient with non-insulin-dependent (type 2) diabetes mellitus produces some insulin and doesn't need exogenous insulin supplementation under normal circumstances. Most patients with this type of diabetes respond well to oral antidiabetic agents, which stimulate the pancreas to increase insulin synthesis and release. **(M-S)**

▶ A patient with insulin-dependent (type 1) diabetes mellitus can't produce endogenous insulin and requires exogenous insulin administration to meet the body's needs. **(M-S)**

▶ Rapid-acting insulins are clear; intermediate- and long-acting insulins are turbid (cloudy). **(M-S)**

▶ Rapid-acting insulins begin to act in 30 to 60 minutes, reach a peak concentration in 2 to 10 hours, and have a duration of action of 5 to 16 hours. **(M-S)**

▶ The best times to test the patient's glucose level are before each meal and at bedtime. **(M-S)**

▶ Intermediate-acting insulins begin to act in 1 to 2 hours, reach a peak concentration in 4 to 15 hours, and have a duration of action of 22 to 28 hours. **(M-S)**

▶ Long-acting insulins begin to act in 4 to 8 hours, reach a peak concentration in 10 to 30 hours, and have a duration of action of 36 or more hours. **(M-S)**

▶ A patient with above-normal glucose levels after glucose administration in a nonfasting glucose test but with normal plasma glucose levels otherwise has impaired glucose tolerance.
(M-S)

▶ Insulin requirements are increased by growth, pregnancy, increased food intake, stress, surgery, infection, illness, increased insulin antibodies, and some medications. **(M-S)**

▶ Insulin requirements are decreased by hypothyroidism, decreased food intake, exercise, and some medications. **(M-S)**

▶ Hypoglycemia occurs when the blood glucose level falls below 50 mg/dl. **(M-S)**

▶ An insulin-resistant patient is one who requires more than 200 U of insulin each day. **(M-S)**

▶ Hypoglycemia may occur 1 to 3 hours after administration of a rapid-acting insulin, 4 to 18 hours after administration of an intermediate-acting insulin, and 18 to 30 hours after administration of a long-acting insulin. **(M-S)**

▶ When the blood glucose level falls rapidly, the patient may experience sweating, tremors, pallor, tachycardia, and palpitations. **(M-S)**

▶ Objective signs of hypoglycemia include slurred speech, lack of coordination, staggered gait, seizures and, possibly, coma. **(M-S)**

▶ A conscious patient with hypoglycemia should receive sugar in a form that can be easily digested, such as orange juice, candy, or lump sugar. **(M-S)**

▶ An unconscious patient with hypoglycemia should receive an S.C. or I.M. injection of glucagon as prescribed by a doctor or 50% dextrose by I.V. injection. **(M-S)**

▶ A patient with diabetes mellitus should inspect the feet daily for calluses, corns, or blisters; wash the feet with warm water; and trim the toenails straight across to prevent ingrown toenails. **(M-S)**

▶ The early stage of ketoacidosis is manifested by polyuria, polydipsia, anorexia, muscle cramps, and vomiting; the late stage is manifested by Kussmaul's respirations, sweet breath odor, and stupor or coma. **(M-S)**

▶ An allergen is a substance capable of producing a hypersensitivity reaction. **(M-S)**

▶ To maintain package sterility, the nurse should open the wrapper's top flap away from the body, open each side flap by touching only the outer part of the wrapper, and open the final flap by grasping the turned-down corner and pulling it toward the body. **(FND)**

▶ A corrective lens for nearsightedness is concave. **(M-S)**

▶ Chronic untreated hypothyroidism or abrupt withdrawal of thyroid medication may lead to myxedema coma.　**(M-S)**

▶ Signs and symptoms of myxedema coma are lethargy, stupor, decreased level of consciousness, dry skin and hair, delayed deep tendon reflexes, progressive respiratory center depression and cerebral hypoxia, weight gain, hypothermia, and hypoglycemia.　**(M-S)**

▶ Nearsightedness occurs when the focal point of a ray of light from an object that is 20′ (6 m) away falls in front of the retina. **(M-S)**

▶ Farsightedness occurs when the focal point of a ray of light from an object that is 20′ (6 m) away falls behind the retina.　**(M-S)**

▶ A corrective lens for farsightedness is convex.　**(M-S)**

▶ Refraction refers to clinical measurement of the error in eye focusing.　**(M-S)**

▶ Adhesions are bands of granulation and scar tissue that develop in some patients after a surgical incision.　**(M-S)**

▶ The nurse should moisten an eye patch for an unconscious patient because a dry patch may irritate the cornea.　**(M-S)**

▶ A patient who has had eye surgery should not bend over, comb the hair vigorously, or engage in activity that increases intraocular pressure.　**(M-S)**

▶ When caring for a patient with a penetrating eye injury, the nurse should loosely patch both eyes with sterile gauze, administer an oral antibiotic (in high doses) and tetanus injection as prescribed, and refer the patient to an ophthalmologist for follow-up.　**(M-S)**

▶ Signs and symptoms of colorectal cancer include changes in bowel habits, rectal bleeding, abdominal pain, anorexia, weight loss, malaise, anemia, and constipation or diarrhea.　**(M-S)**

▶ When climbing stairs with crutches, the patient should lead with the uninvolved leg and follow with the crutches and involved leg.　**(M-S)**

► When descending stairs with crutches, the patient should lead with the crutches and the involved leg and follow with the uninvolved leg. **(M-S)**

► When surgery requires eyelash trimming, the nurse should apply petroleum jelly to the scissor blades so that the eyelashes will adhere to them. **(M-S)**

► Pain after a corneal transplant may indicate that the dressing has been applied too tightly, the graft has slipped, or the eye is hemorrhaging. **(M-S)**

► A patient with retinal detachment may report floating spots, flashes of light, and a sensation of a veil or curtain coming down. **(M-S)**

► Immediate postoperative care for a patient with retinal detachment includes maintaining the eye patch and shield in place over the affected area and observing for drainage; maintaining the patient in the position specified by the ophthalmologist (usually the patient is lying on his abdomen, with his head parallel to the floor and turned to the side); avoiding bumping the patient's head or bed; and encouraging deep breathing but not coughing. **(M-S)**

► A patient with a cataract may report vision disturbances, such as image distortion, light glaring, and gradual loss of vision. **(M-S)**

► When talking to a hearing impaired patient who can lip-read, the nurse should speak slowly and enunciate clearly, point to objects as needed, avoid chewing gum, and face the patient. **(M-S)**

► Clinical manifestations of venous stasis ulcer include hemosiderin deposits (visible in fair-skinned individuals), dry cracked skin, and infection. **(M-S)**

► The fluorescent treponemal antibody absorption test is a specific serologic test for syphilis. **(M-S)**

► The nurse may use a sponge bath with tepid water (80° to 93° F [27° to 34° C]) to reduce fever. **(M-S)**

▶ When communicating with a patient who has had a cerebrovascular accident, the nurse should allow ample time for the patient to speak and respond, face the patient's unaffected side, avoid talking fast, give visual clues, supplement speech with gestures, and give instructions consistently. **(M-S)**

▶ The major complication of Bell's palsy is keratitis (corneal inflammation), which results from incomplete eye closure on the affected side. **(M-S)**

▶ Immunosuppressants are used to combat tissue rejection and help control autoimmune disorders. **(M-S)**

▶ After a unilateral cerebrovascular accident, a patient may be able to propel a wheelchair by using a heel-to-toe movement with the unaffected leg and turning the wheel with the unaffected hand. **(M-S)**

▶ First-morning urine is the most concentrated and most likely to reveal abnormalities. It should be refrigerated to retard bacterial growth or, for microscopic examination, should be sent to the laboratory immediately. **(M-S)**

▶ The patient recovering from a cerebrovascular accident should align the arms and legs correctly, wear high-top sneakers to prevent footdrop and contracture, and use an egg crate, flotation, or pulsating mattress to help prevent pressure ulcers. **(M-S)**

▶ After an arm or leg fracture, the bone may display complete union (normal healing), delayed union (healing that takes longer than expected), or nonunion (failure to heal). **(M-S)**

▶ The most common complication of a hip fracture is thromboembolism, which may occlude an artery and cause the area it supplies to become cold and cyanotic. **(M-S)**

▶ Chloral hydrate suppositories should be refrigerated. **(M-S)**

▶ Cast application usually requires two persons; it shouldn't be attempted alone. **(M-S)**

▶ A plaster cast reaches maximum strength in 48 hours; a synthetic cast, within 30 minutes because it doesn't require drying.
(M-S)

▶ Severe pain indicates pressure ulcer development within a cast; the pain decreases significantly once an ulcer develops. **(M-S)**

▶ With running traction (Buck's traction), the patient may not be turned without disrupting the line of pull; with balanced suspension traction, the patient may be elevated, turned slightly, and moved as needed. **(PED)**

▶ Indications of circulatory interference are abnormal skin coolness, cyanosis, and rubor or pallor. **(M-S)**

▶ During the postoperative phase, a rising pulse rate and falling blood pressure may indicate hemorrhage and impending shock. **(M-S)**

▶ Orthopedic surgical wounds bleed more than other surgical wounds. The nurse can expect 200 to 500 ml of drainage during the first 24 hours and less than 30 ml each 8 hours for the next 48 hours. **(M-S)**

▶ A patient who has had hip surgery shouldn't adduct or flex the operated hip because flexion greater than 90 degrees may cause dislocation. **(M-S)**

▶ The Hoyer lift, a hydraulic device, enables two persons to lift and move a nonambulatory patient safely. **(M-S)**

▶ A patient with carpal tunnel syndrome, a complex of symptoms caused by median nerve compression in the carpal tunnel, usually reports weakness, pain, burning, numbness, or tingling in one or both hands. **(M-S)**

▶ The nurse shouldn't use a cotton-tipped applicator to dry a patient's ear canal or remove wax because it may force cerumen against the tympanic membrane. **(FND)**

▶ Hyperalertness is a symptom of posttraumatic stress disorder.
(PSY)

▶ A patient's identification bracelet should remain in place until the patient has been discharged from the health care facility and has left the premises. **(FND)**

▶ The nurse should instruct a patient who has had heatstroke to wear light-colored, loose-fitting clothing when exposed to the sun; rest frequently; and drink plenty of fluids. **(M-S)**

▶ A conscious patient with heat exhaustion or heatstroke should receive a solution of ½ teaspoon of salt in 120 ml of water every 15 minutes for 1 hour. **(M-S)**

▶ An I.V. line inserted during an emergency or outside the hospital setting should be changed within 24 hours. **(M-S)**

▶ The nurse should discontinue the tepid bath and notify the doctor if the patient develops cyanosis or a change in pulse rate or respirations. **(M-S)**

▶ After a tepid bath, the nurse should dry the patient thoroughly to prevent chills. **(M-S)**

▶ The nurse should take the patient's temperature 30 minutes after completing a tepid bath. **(M-S)**

▶ Shower or bath water shouldn't exceed 105° F (40.5° C). **(M-S)**

▶ Dilatation and curettage is the widening of the cervical canal with a dilator and the scraping of the uterus with a curette. **(M-S)**

▶ When not in use, all central venous catheters must be capped with adaptors after flushing. **(M-S)**

▶ Care after a dilatation and curettage consists of bed rest for 1 day, mild analgesics for pain, and use of a sterile pad for as long as bleeding persists. **(M-S)**

▶ If a patient feels faint during a bath or shower, the nurse should turn off the water, cover the patient, lower the patient's head, and summon help. **(M-S)**

▶ For the first few months of levothyroxine sodium (Synthroid) therapy, a child may experience temporary hair loss.   **(PED)**

▶ A patient taking oral contraceptives shouldn't smoke because smoking can intensify the drug's adverse cardiovascular effect.
(M-S)

▶ The use of soft restraints requires a doctor's order as well as assessment and documentation of the patient and affected limbs, according to facility policy.   **(M-S)**

▶ A vest restraint should be used cautiously in a patient with heart failure or a respiratory disorder because it can tighten with movement, further limiting respiratory function. Also, the least amount of restraint should be used to ensure patient safety.
(M-S)

▶ If a piggyback system becomes dislodged, the nurse should replace the entire piggyback system with the appropriate solution and medication as prescribed.   **(M-S)**

▶ The nurse shouldn't secure a restraint to the bed's side rails because they might be inadvertently lowered, causing patient injury or discomfort.   **(M-S)**

▶ Before discharging a patient who has had an abortion, the nurse should instruct her to report bright red clots, bleeding that lasts longer than 7 days, or signs of infection, such as a temperature above 100° F (37.8° C), foul-smelling vaginal discharge, severe uterine cramping, nausea, or vomiting.   **(MAT)**

▶ The nurse should assess a patient with limb restraints every 30 minutes to detect signs of impaired circulation.   **(M-S)**

▶ The Centers for Disease Control and Prevention recommends using a needleless system for piggybacking an I.V. medication into the main I.V. line.   **(M-S)**

▶ When informed that a patient's amniotic membrane has broken, the nurse should first check fetal heart tones and then maternal vital signs.   **(MAT)**

▶ A mask should be replaced every 30 minutes.   **(M-S)**

▶ If a gown is required, the nurse should put it on upon entering the patient's room and discard it upon leaving. **(M-S)**

▶ When changing the dressing of a patient in isolation, the nurse should wear two pairs of gloves. **(M-S)**

▶ The duration of pregnancy averages 280 days, 40 weeks, 9 calendar months, or 10 lunar months. **(MAT)**

▶ A disposable bedpan and urinal should remain in the room of a patient in isolation and be discarded on discharge or at the end of the isolation period. **(M-S)**

▶ Mycoses (fungal infections) may be systemic or deep (affecting the internal organs), subcutaneous (involving the skin), or superficial (growing on the outer layer of skin and hair). **(M-S)**

▶ The night before a sputum specimen is to be collected by expectoration, the patient should increase fluid intake to promote sputum production. **(M-S)**

▶ A stool sample for an ova and parasite study should be collected directly into a waterproof container, covered with a lid, and sent immediately to the laboratory. If the patient is bedridden, the sample can be collected into a clean, dry bedpan and then transferred with a tongue depressor into a container. **(M-S)**

▶ When obtaining a sputum specimen for testing, the nurse should instruct the patient to rinse the mouth with clean water, cough deeply from the chest, and expectorate into a sterile container. **(M-S)**

▶ Tonometry allows indirect measurement of intraocular pressure and aids in early detection of glaucoma. **(M-S)**

▶ Pulmonary function tests (a series of measurements that evaluate ventilatory function through spirometric measurements) help diagnose pulmonary dysfunction. **(M-S)**

▶ After a liver biopsy, the patient should lie on the right side to compress the biopsy site, which decreases the possibility of bleeding. **(M-S)**

► A patient with cirrhosis should follow a diet that restricts sodium but provides protein, vitamins (especially B, C, and K and folate), and at least 3,000 calories a day.   **(M-S)**

► If 12 hours of gastric suction don't relieve bowel obstruction, surgery is indicated.   **(M-S)**

► The nurse can puncture a nifedipine (Procardia) capsule with a needle, withdraw its liquid, and instill it into the buccal pouch.   **(M-S)**

► When administering whole blood or packed red blood cells (RBCs), the nurse should use a 16G to 20G needle or cannula to avoid RBC hemolysis.   **(M-S)**

► Hirsutism is excessive body hair in a masculine distribution.   **(M-S)**

► The Controlled Substances Act designated five categories, or schedules, that classify controlled drugs according to their abuse liability.   **(FND)**

► Schedule I drugs, such as heroin, have a high abuse potential and have no currently accepted medical use in the United States.   **(FND)**

► Schedule II drugs, such as morphine, opium, and meperidine (Demerol), have a high abuse potential but have currently accepted medical uses. Their use may lead to physical or psychological dependence.   **(FND)**

► Schedule III drugs, such as paregoric and butabarbital (Butisol), have a lower abuse potential than Schedule I or II drugs. Abuse of Schedule III drugs may lead to moderate or low physical or psychological dependence, or both.   **(FND)**

► Schedule IV drugs, such as chloral hydrate, have a low abuse potential compared with Schedule III drugs.   **(FND)**

► Schedule V drugs, such as cough syrups that contain codeine, have the lowest abuse potential of the controlled substances.   **(FND)**

▶ One unit of whole blood or packed red blood cells should be administered over 2 to 4 hours. **(M-S)**

▶ For I.V. medication administration in an infant or an older patient with small veins, the nurse should use a 21G or 23G winged set, dilute the medication as prescribed, and infuse it slowly to prevent vein injury. **(PED)**

▶ Scurvy is associated with vitamin C deficiency. **(M-S)**

▶ A vitamin is an organic compound that usually can't be synthesized by the body and is needed in metabolic processes. **(M-S)**

▶ An adolescent's eating habits are significantly influenced by the peer group. **(PED)**

▶ In an infant, manifestations of hypothyroidism are inactivity, excessive sleeping, and minimal crying (and the infant may be described as a "good baby"). **(PED)**

▶ Pulmonary embolism can be caused by thromboembolism of fat, blood, bone marrow, or amniotic fluid obstructing the pulmonary artery. **(M-S)**

▶ After maxillofacial surgery, a patient whose mandible and maxilla have been wired together should keep a pair of scissors or wire cutters readily available to prevent aspiration if vomiting occurs and the wires need to be cut. **(M-S)**

▶ Rapid instillation of fluid during colonic irrigation can cause abdominal cramping. **(M-S)**

▶ A collaborative environment between health care workers helps shorten the hospital stay and increase patient satisfaction. **(M-S)**

▶ Predictable hazards for elderly patients in a health care facility include nighttime confusion (sundowning), fractures from falling, immobility-induced pressure ulcers, prolonged convalescence, and loss of home and support systems. **(M-S)**

▶ Respiratory tract infections—especially viral ones—can trigger asthma attacks. **(M-S)**

▶ Oxygen therapy is used in severe asthma attacks to prevent or treat hypoxemia. **(M-S)**

▶ During an asthma attack, the patient may prefer nasal prongs to a Venturi mask because of the mask's smothering effect. **(M-S)**

▶ Chronic obstructive pulmonary disease usually develops over a period of years and results from smoking in 95% of patients. **(M-S)**

▶ An early sign of chronic obstructive pulmonary disease (COPD) is slowing of forced expiration. A healthy person can empty the lungs in less than 4 seconds; a patient with COPD may take 6 to 10 seconds. **(M-S)**

▶ Chronic obstructive pulmonary disease eventually leads to structural changes in the lungs, including overdistended alveoli and hyperinflated lungs. **(M-S)**

▶ Cystic fibrosis, which is transmitted as an autosomal recessive trait, causes dysfunction of the exocrine gland, sweat glands, and respiratory and digestive systems. **(PED)**

▶ A common manifestation of cystic fibrosis in the newborn is meconium ileus caused by obstruction of the small intestine by viscous meconium. **(PED)**

▶ Infants who have cystic fibrosis but don't have meconium ileus at birth have good appetites but gain weight slowly. **(PED)**

▶ Cellulitis is manifested as localized heat, redness, swelling and, occasionally, fever, chills, and malaise. **(M-S)**

▶ The initial weight loss for a healthy neonate is 5% to 10% of the birth weight. **(MAT)**

▶ The hemoglobin value in neonates normally ranges from 17 to 20 g/dl. **(MAT)**

▶ Venous stasis may precipitate thrombophlebitis. **(M-S)**

▶ Thrombophlebitis treatment includes leg elevation, heat application and, possibly, anticoagulant therapy. **(M-S)**

▶ A suctioning machine should remain at the bedside of a patient who has had maxillofacial surgery. **(M-S)**

▶ For a bedridden patient with heart failure, the nurse should check for edema in the sacral area. **(M-S)**

▶ Crowning describes the appearance of the fetus's head when its largest diameter is encircled by the vulvovaginal ring.

(MAT)

▶ If an immunization schedule is interrupted for any reason, it should be restarted from the last immunization administered and not from the beginning. **(PED)**

▶ In passive range-of-motion exercises, the therapist moves the patient's joints through as full a range of motion as possible to improve or maintain joint mobility and help prevent contractures. **(M-S)**

▶ In resistance exercises, which allow muscle length to change, the patient performs exercises against resistance applied by the therapist. **(M-S)**

▶ In isometric exercises, the patient contracts muscles against stable resistance but without joint movement. The muscle length remains the same, but muscle strength and tone may increase. **(M-S)**

▶ Predisposing factors for impetigo (a contagious, superficial, vesicopustular skin infection) include poor hygiene, anemia, malnutrition, and a warm climate. **(M-S)**

▶ Activities of daily living are actions that the patient must perform every day to provide self-care and interact with society.

(FND)

▶ After cardiopulmonary resuscitation (CPR) begins, it shouldn't be interrupted, except when a rescuer is alone and must summon help. In such a case, the rescuer should perform CPR for 1 minute before calling for help. **(M-S)**

▶ The tongue is the most common airway obstruction in an unconscious patient. **(M-S)**

▶ For adult cardiopulmonary resuscitation, the chest compression rate is 80 to 100 times per minute. **(M-S)**

▶ A patient with ulcers should avoid bedtime snacks because food may stimulate nocturnal secretions. **(M-S)**

▶ In angioplasty, a blood vessel is dilated by a balloon catheter inserted through the skin and the vessel's lumen to the narrowed area. Once in place, the balloon is inflated to flatten plaque against the vessel wall. **(M-S)**

▶ A full liquid diet supplies nutrients, fluids, and calories in simple, easily digested foods, such as apple juice, cream of wheat, milk, coffee, strained cream soup, high-protein gelatin, cranberry juice, custard, and ice cream. It is prescribed for patients who can't tolerate a regular diet. **(M-S)**

▶ A pureed diet meets the patient's nutritional needs without foods that are difficult for the patient to chew or swallow. Food is blended to a semisolid consistency. **(M-S)**

▶ A soft, or light, diet is specifically designed for patients who have difficulty chewing or tolerating a regular diet. It is nutritionally adequate and consists of foods such as orange juice, cream of wheat, scrambled eggs, enriched toast, cream of chicken soup, wheat bread, fruit cocktail, and mushroom soup. **(M-S)**

▶ A regular diet is provided for patients who don't require any dietary modification. **(M-S)**

▶ A pediatric diet normally is ordered as "diet for age" by the doctor. It should include sufficient nutrients and calories to promote growth and development. **(PED)**

▶ A bland diet restricts foods that cause gastric irritation or produce acid secretion without providing a neutralizing effect. **(M-S)**

▶ A clear liquid diet provides fluid and a gradual return to a regular diet; however, it is deficient in all nutrients, and the patient should consume this diet for only a short period. **(M-S)**

▶ Patients with a gastric ulcer should avoid alcohol, caffeinated beverages, aspirin, and spicy foods. **(M-S)**

▶ In active assistance exercises, the patient performs exercises with the therapist's help. **(M-S)**

▶ Penicillinase is an enzyme produced by certain bacteria. It converts penicillin into an inactive product, thereby increasing the bacteria's resistance to the antibiotic. **(M-S)**

▶ Battle's sign is a bluish discoloration behind the ear in some patients who sustain a basilar skull fracture. **(M-S)**

▶ Crackles are nonmusical clicking or rattling noises heard during auscultation of abnormal breath sounds. They result from air passing through fluid-filled airways. **(M-S)**

▶ Antibiotics aren't effective against viruses, protozoa, or parasites. **(M-S)**

▶ Most penicillins and cephalosporins produce their antibiotic effects by cell wall inhibition. **(M-S)**

▶ When assessing a patient with an inguinal hernia, the nurse should suspect strangulation if the patient reports severe pain, nausea, and vomiting. **(M-S)**

▶ Phimosis is tightness of the prepuce of the penis that prevents foreskin retraction over the glans. **(M-S)**

▶ Aminoglycosides are natural antibiotics that are effective against gram-negative bacteria. They must be used with caution because they can cause nephrotoxicity and ototoxicity.
(M-S)

▶ Upon scrotal examination, varicoceles and tumors don't transilluminate, but spermatoceles and hydroceles do. **(M-S)**

▶ The heart of a child with tetralogy of Fallot appears boot-shaped on X-ray films because the right ventricle is enlarged.
(PED)

▶ Testing of the six cardinal fields of gaze evaluates the function of all extraocular muscles and cranial nerves III, IV, and VI.
(FND)

▶ A hordeolum (eyelid stye) represents an infection of one or more sebaceous glands of the eyelid.   **(M-S)**

▶ A chalazion is an eyelid mass that results from chronic inflammation of the meibomian gland.   **(M-S)**

▶ During an ophthalmoscopic examination, the absence of the red reflex indicates a lens opacity (cataract) or a detached retina.
(M-S)

▶ Respiratory acidosis is associated with conditions such as drug overdose, Guillain-Barré syndrome, myasthenia gravis, chronic obstructive pulmonary disease, pickwickian syndrome, and kyphoscoliosis.   **(M-S)**

▶ Respiratory alkalosis is associated with conditions such as high fever, severe hypoxia, asthma, and pulmonary embolism.
(M-S)

▶ Metabolic acidosis is associated with conditions such as renal failure, diarrhea, diabetic ketosis, and lactic ketosis and with high doses of acetazolamide (Diamox).   **(M-S)**

▶ Gastrectomy is the surgical excision of all or part of the stomach to remove a chronic peptic ulcer, to stop hemorrhage in the perforated ulcer, or to remove a malignant tumor.   **(M-S)**

▶ Metabolic alkalosis is associated with nasogastric suctioning, excessive diuretic use, and steroid therapy.   **(M-S)**

▶ Vitiligo (a benign, acquired skin disease) is marked by stark-white skin patches resulting from the destruction and loss of pigment cells.   **(M-S)**

▶ A multipara is a woman who has had two or more pregnancies that progressed to viability (whether or not the offspring were alive at birth).   **(MAT)**

▶ Overdose or accidental overingestion of disulfiram (Antabuse) should be treated by gastric aspiration or lavage along with supportive therapy. **(M-S)**

▶ The six types of heart murmurs are graded from 1 to 6. A grade 6 heart murmur can be heard with the stethoscope slightly raised from the chest. **(FND)**

▶ The causes of abdominal distention are represented by the six *F's:* flatus, feces, fetus, fluid, fat, and fatal (malignant) neoplasm. **(M-S)**

▶ A positive Murphy's sign indicates cholecystitis. **(M-S)**

▶ Signs of appendicitis include right abdominal pain, abdominal rigidity and rebound tenderness, nausea, and anorexia. **(M-S)**

▶ Ascites can be detected when more than 500 ml of fluid has collected in the intraperitoneal space. **(M-S)**

▶ The most important goal to include in a care plan is the patient's goal. **(FND)**

▶ The ideal environment for a patient with organic brain syndrome or a senile disease is one that is stable and limits confusion. **(M-S)**

▶ Memory loss in organic brain syndrome usually affects all spheres but begins with recent memory loss. **(M-S)**

▶ In a pregnant patient, preeclampsia may progress to eclampsia, which is characterized by seizures and may lead to coma. **(MAT)**

▶ The nurse assigns an Apgar score to a neonate at 1 and 5 minutes after birth. The score is based on respiratory effort, heart rate, muscle tone, reflex irritability, and color. **(MAT)**

▶ During cardiac catheterization, the patient may experience a thudding sensation in the chest, a strong desire to cough, and a transient feeling of heat, usually in the face, from the contrast medium injection. **(M-S)**

► Insulin requirements increase during the third trimester because of the anti-insulin effects of placental hormones. **(MAT)**

► Gestational age can be estimated by ultrasound measurement of abdominal circumference, femur length, and fetal head size. Such measurements are most accurate between 12 and 18 weeks' gestation. **(MAT)**

► Skeletal system abnormalities and ventricular septal defects are the most common disorders of infants born to diabetic women. The incidence of congenital malformation is three times higher in these infants than in those born to nondiabetic women. **(MAT)**

► Slight bubbling in the suction column of a thoracic drainage system such as a Pleur-evac unit indicates that it's working properly; a lack of bubbling in the suction chamber indicates inadequate suction. **(M-S)**

► Nutritional deficiency is a common finding in people who have a long history of alcohol abuse. **(M-S)**

► Treatment for alcohol withdrawal may include administration of I.V. glucose for hypoglycemia, I.V. fluid containing thiamine and other B vitamins, and antianxiety, antidiarrheal, anticonvulsant, and antiemetic drugs. **(PSY)**

► The alcoholic patient receives thiamine to help prevent peripheral neuropathy and Korsakoff's syndrome. **(PSY)**

► Alcohol withdrawal may precipitate seizure activity because alcohol lowers the seizure threshold in some people. **(PSY)**

► Paraphrasing is an active listening technique in which the nurse restates what the patient has just conveyed. **(PSY)**

► The patient with Korsakoff's syndrome may use confabulation (made up information) to cover memory lapses or periods of amnesia. **(PSY)**

► Graduated compression elastic stockings (30 to 40 mm Hg) may be prescribed to promote venous return in the patient with varicose veins. **(M-S)**

▶ Nonviral hepatitis usually results from exposure to certain chemicals or drugs. **(M-S)**

▶ The patient with preeclampsia usually complains of puffiness around the eyes or edema in the hands (for example, "I can't put my wedding ring on."). **(MAT)**

▶ A symptom of acute hepatitis is a substantial elevation of the serum transaminase level. **(M-S)**

▶ Normal cardiac output is 4 to 6 L/minute with a stroke volume of 60 to 70 ml. **(M-S)**

▶ Excessive vomiting or removal of stomach contents through suction can decrease the potassium level and lead to hypokalemia. **(M-S)**

▶ As a heparin antagonist, protamine sulfate is an antidote for heparin overdose. **(M-S)**

▶ People with obsessive-compulsive disorder realize that their behavior is unreasonable but are powerless to control it. **(PSY)**

▶ If the patient has a positive reaction to a tuberculin skin test, such as the purified protein derivative test, the nurse should suspect current or past exposure and should ask about a history of tuberculosis (TB) and the presence of early signs and symptoms of TB, such as low-grade fever, weight loss, night sweats, fatigue, and anorexia. **(M-S)**

▶ Signs and symptoms of acute rheumatic fever include chorea, fever, carditis, migratory polyarthritis, erythema marginatum (rash), and subcutaneous nodules. **(M-S)**

▶ The patient with a history of rheumatic fever should receive prophylactic penicillin therapy before undergoing any invasive procedure to help prevent blood contamination with oral bacteria, which could migrate to the heart valves. **(M-S)**

▶ Fruits are high in fiber and low in protein and should be omitted from a low-residue diet. **(FND)**

▶ The nurse should use an objective scale to assess and quantify pain because postoperative pain varies greatly among individuals. **(FND)**

▶ After a myocardial infarction, most patients can resume sexual activity when they can climb two flights of stairs without fatigue or dyspnea. **(M-S)**

▶ Elderly patients are susceptible to orthostatic hypotension because with age the baroreceptors become less sensitive to position changes. **(M-S)**

▶ Kegel exercises require contraction and relaxation of the perineal muscles to help strengthen pelvic muscles and improve urine control in postpartum patients. **(MAT)**

▶ When witnessing psychiatric patients in a threatening confrontation, the nurse should first separate the two individuals. **(PSY)**

▶ Symptoms of postpartum depression range from mild postpartum blues to an intense, suicidal, depressive psychosis. **(MAT)**

▶ The preterm neonate may require gavage feedings because of a weak sucking reflex, uncoordinated sucking, or respiratory distress. **(MAT)**

▶ Postmortem care includes cleaning and preparing the deceased patient for family viewing, arranging transportation to the morgue or funeral home, and determining the disposition of belongings. **(FND)**

▶ For the patient with suspected renal or urethral calculi, the nurse should strain the urine to determine if calculi have been passed. **(M-S)**

▶ The nurse should place the patient with ascites in semi-Fowler's position because it affords maximum lung expansion. **(M-S)**

▶ For the patient who has ingested poison, the nurse should save the vomitus for analysis. **(M-S)**

▶ The nurse should provide honest answers to the patient's questions. **(FND)**

▶ Acrocyanosis (blueness and coolness of the arms and legs) is normal in neonates because of their immature peripheral circulatory system. **(MAT)**

▶ The earliest signs of respiratory distress are increased respiratory rate followed by increased pulse rate. **(M-S)**

▶ In adults, gastroenteritis usually is self-limiting and produces diarrhea, abdominal discomfort, nausea, and vomiting. **(M-S)**

▶ Cardiac output equals stroke volume multiplied by the heart rate per minute. **(M-S)**

▶ Milk shouldn't be included in a clear liquid diet. **(FND)**

▶ In patients with acute meningitis, the cerebrospinal fluid protein level is elevated. **(M-S)**

▶ When the patient is suspected of having food poisoning, the nurse should notify public health authorities so they can interview patients and food handlers and take samples of the suspected contaminated food. **(M-S)**

▶ The patient receiving a potassium-wasting diuretic should eat potassium-rich foods. **(M-S)**

▶ Consistency in nursing personnel is paramount when caring for a child, an infant, or a confused patient. **(FND)**

▶ The patient with chronic obstructive pulmonary disease should receive low level oxygen by nasal cannula (2 to 3 L/minute) so as not to interfere with their hypoxic drive. **(M-S)**

▶ The hypothalamus secretes vasopressin and oxytocin, which are stored in the pituitary gland. **(FND)**

▶ The three membranes that enclose the brain and spinal cord are the dura mater, pia mater, and arachnoid. **(FND)**

▶ A nasogastric tube is used to remove fluid and gas from the small intestine preoperatively or postoperatively. **(FND)**

▶ To prevent ophthalmia neonatorum (a severe eye infection caused by maternal gonorrhea), the nurse may administer one of three medications, as prescribed, in the neonate's eyes: tetracycline, silver nitrate, or erythromycin.   **(MAT)**

▶ In metabolic acidosis, the patient may develop Kussmaul's respirations because the rate and depth of respirations increase to "blow off" excess carbonic acids.   **(M-S)**

▶ In a female patient, gonorrhea affects the vagina and fallopian tubes.   **(M-S)**

▶ Phenylketonuria is an inborn error in phenylalanine metabolism, resulting in high serum levels of phenylalanine that might cause cerebral damage and mental retardation.   **(PED)**

▶ The greatest threats to the patient who has suffered traumatic amputation are blood loss and hypovolemic shock; thus, initial interventions should control bleeding and replace fluid and blood as needed.   **(M-S)**

▶ Epinephrine is a sympathomimetic drug that acts primarily on alpha, $beta_1$, and $beta_2$ receptors, causing vasoconstriction.   **(M-S)**

▶ Epinephrine's adverse effects include dyspnea, tachycardia, palpitations, headaches, and hypertension.   **(M-S)**

▶ Psychologists, physical therapists, and chiropractors aren't authorized to write prescriptions for medication.   **(FND)**

▶ The area around a stoma should be cleaned with mild soap and water.   **(FND)**

▶ Vegetables have a high fiber content.   **(FND)**

▶ A cardinal sign of pancreatitis is an elevated serum amylase level.   **(M-S)**

▶ High colonic irrigation is used to stimulate peristalsis and reduce flatulence.   **(M-S)**

▶ The nurse should use a tuberculin syringe to administer an S.C. injection of less than 1 ml.   **(FND)**

▶ Bleeding is the most common postoperative problem. **(M-S)**

▶ The patient can control some colostomy odors by not eating such foods as fish, eggs, onions, beans, and cabbages and related vegetables. **(M-S)**

▶ For adults, S.C. injections require a 25G 1″ needle; for infants, children, elderly, or very thin patients, they require a 25G to 27G ½″ needle. **(FND)**

▶ Before administering medication, the nurse should identify the patient by checking the identification band and asking the patient to state his name. **(FND)**

▶ To clean the skin before an injection, the nurse should use a sterile alcohol swab and wipe from the center of the site outward in a circular motion. **(FND)**

▶ The nurse always should inject heparin deep into S.C. tissue at a 90-degree angle (perpendicular to the skin) to prevent skin irritation. **(FND)**

▶ If blood is aspirated into the syringe before an I.M. injection, the nurse should withdraw the needle, prepare another syringe, and repeat the procedure. **(FND)**

▶ The nurse shouldn't cut the patient's hair without written consent from the patient or an appropriate relative. **(FND)**

▶ If bleeding occurs after an injection, the nurse should apply pressure until the bleeding stops; if bruising occurs, the nurse should monitor the site for an enlarging hematoma. **(FND)**

▶ When providing hair and scalp care, the nurse should begin combing at the end of the hair and work toward the head. **(FND)**

▶ Frequency of patient hair care depends on the length and texture of the hair, duration of hospitalization, and patient's condition. **(FND)**

▶ When paralysis or coma impairs or erases the corneal reflex, frequent eye care is designed to keep the exposed cornea moist, preventing ulceration and inflammation. **(M-S)**

▶ Proper hearing aid function requires careful handling during insertion and removal, regular cleaning of the ear piece to prevent wax buildup, and prompt replacement of dead batteries. **(FND)**

▶ The hearing aid marked with a blue dot is for the left ear; the one with the red dot is for the right ear. **(FND)**

▶ A hearing aid shouldn't be exposed to heat or humidity and shouldn't be immersed in water. **(FND)**

▶ The nurse should instruct a patient not to use hair spray while wearing a hearing aid. **(FND)**

▶ The five branches of pharmacology are pharmacokinetics, pharmacodynamics, pharmacotherapeutics, toxicology, and pharmacognosy. **(FND)**

▶ Interventions for the patient with acquired immunodeficiency syndrome include treating existing infections and cancers, reducing the risk of opportunistic infections, maintaining adequate nutrition and hydration, and providing emotional support to the patient and family. **(M-S)**

▶ The nurse should remove heel protectors every 8 hours to inspect the foot for signs of skin breakdown. **(FND)**

▶ Signs and symptoms of a chlamydial infection are urinary frequency; thin, white vaginal or urethral discharge; and cervical inflammation. **(M-S)**

▶ The purpose of heat application is to promote vasodilation, which reduces pain caused by inflammation. **(FND)**

▶ Chlamydial infection is the most prevalent sexually transmitted disease in the United States. **(M-S)**

▶ The pituitary gland is located in the sella turcica of the sphenoid bone in the cranial cavity. **(M-S)**

▶ Myasthenia gravis is a neuromuscular disorder characterized by impulse disturbances at the myoneural junction. **(M-S)**

▶ A sutured surgical incision is an example of healing by first intention (healing directly, without granulation). **(FND)**

▶ Healing by secondary intention (healing by granulation) is closure of the wound by the granulation tissue filling the defect and allowing reepithelialization to occur, beginning at the wound edges and continuing to the center, until the entire wound is covered. **(FND)**

▶ Keloid formation is an abnormality in healing characterized by overgrowth of scar tissue at the wound site. **(FND)**

▶ Patients with anorexia nervosa or bulimia must be observed during the meal and for a time afterward to ensure that they don't purge what they have eaten. **(PSY)**

▶ Myasthenia gravis usually affects young women, producing extreme muscle weakness and fatigability, difficulty chewing and talking, strabismus, and ptosis. **(M-S)**

▶ Transsexuals believe that they were born the wrong gender and may seek hormonal or surgical treatment to change their gender. **(PSY)**

▶ Tay-Sachs disease results from a congenital enzyme deficiency and is characterized by progressive mental and motor deterioration and cherry-red spots on the macula. **(PED)**

▶ Hypothermia is a life-threatening disorder in which the body's core temperature drops below 95° F (35° C). **(M-S)**

▶ Treatment of phenylketonuria must begin within the first few weeks of life to prevent brain damage. **(PED)**

▶ Neonatal testing for phenylketonuria has become mandatory in most states. **(MAT)**

▶ Although no cure exists for Tay-Sachs disease, serum analysis for hexosaminidase A deficiency allows for accurate identification of genetic carriers of the disease. **(PED)**

▶ Signs and symptoms of hypopituitarism in adults may include gonadal failure, diabetes insipidus, hypothyroidism, and adrenocortical insufficiency. **(M-S)**

▶ Reiter's syndrome causes a triad of symptoms: arthritis, conjunctivitis, and urethritis. **(M-S)**

▶ Down syndrome (trisomy 21) is the most common chromosomal disorder. **(PED)**

▶ A carbohydrate-restricted diet for patients who have had a partial gastrectomy provides foods high in protein and fats and restricts foods high in carbohydrates because they are quickly digested and are more readily emptied from the stomach into the duodenum, causing diarrhea and dumping syndrome. **(M-S)**

▶ The nurse should place the neonate in a 30-degree Trendelenburg position to facilitate mucus drainage. **(MAT)**

▶ The nurse may suction the neonate's nose and mouth as needed with a bulb syringe or suction trap. **(MAT)**

▶ To prevent heat loss, the nurse first should place the neonate under a radiant warmer during suctioning and initial delivery-room care and then should wrap the neonate in a warmed blanket for transport to the nursery. **(MAT)**

▶ The umbilical cord normally has two arteries and one vein. **(MAT)**

▶ When providing care, the nurse should expose only one part of an infant's body at a time. **(MAT)**

▶ Lightening is the settling of the fetal head into the brim of the pelvis. **(MAT)**

▶ If the neonate is stable, the mother should be allowed to breastfeed within the neonate's first hour of life. **(MAT)**

▶ The nurse should check the neonate's temperature every 1 to 2 hours until it is maintained within normal limits. **(MAT)**

▶ At birth, the neonate normally weighs 5 to 9 lb (2.3 to 4.1 kg), measures 18″ to 22″ (45.7 to 55.9 cm) in length, has a head circumference of 13½″ to 14″ (34.3 to 35.6 cm), and has a chest circumference that is 1″ (2.5 cm) less than the head circumference. **(MAT)**

▶ In the neonate, temperature normally ranges from 98° to 99° F (36.7° to 37.2° C), apical pulse rate averages 120 to 160 beats/minute, and respirations are 40 to 60 breaths/minute. **(MAT)**

▶ The diamond-shaped anterior fontanel usually closes between ages 12 and 18 months; the triangular posterior fontanel usually closes by age 2 months. **(MAT)**

▶ In the neonate, a straight spine is normal; a tuft of hair over the spine is an abnormal finding. **(MAT)**

▶ Prostaglandin gel may be applied to the vagina or cervix to ripen an unfavorable cervix before labor induction with oxytocin (Pitocin). **(MAT)**

▶ When administering an oral medication to an infant, the nurse should place it in the side of the mouth and encourage swallowing by gently lifting the infant's chin with the thumb and stroking the infant's neck. **(PED)**

▶ Supernumerary nipples occasionally are seen on neonates and usually appear along a line that runs from each axilla through the normal nipple area to the groin. **(MAT)**

▶ Meconium is a material that collects in the fetus's intestines and forms the neonate's first stools, which are black and tarry. **(MAT)**

▶ The presence of meconium in the amniotic fluid during labor indicates possible fetal distress and the need to evaluate the neonate for meconium aspiration. **(MAT)**

▶ Polydactyly (more than the normal number of fingers or toes) is a congenital anomaly. **(PED)**

▶ A positive Babinski's reflex (toe fanning when the sole is stroked from heel to toe) is normal in the neonate and may persist for up to 18 months. **(PED)**

▶ To assess the rooting reflex, the nurse touches a finger to the neonate's cheek or corner of mouth. Normally, the neonate turns his head toward the stimulus, opens the mouth, and searches for the stimulus. **(MAT)**

▶ Harlequin sign is present when the neonate lying on the side appears red on the dependent side and pale on the upper side. **(MAT)**

▶ The nurse should administer procaine penicillin by deep I.M. injection in the upper outer portion of the buttocks in the adult or in the midlateral thigh in the child. The nurse shouldn't massage the injection site. **(FND)**

▶ Mongolian spots are slight gray patches across the sacrum, buttocks, and legs. These normal blue-green variations are common in non-white infants and usually disappear by age 2 to 3. **(MAT)**

▶ Vernix caseosa is a cheeselike substance that covers and protects the fetus's skin in utero. It may be rubbed into the neonate's skin or washed away in one or two baths. **(MAT)**

▶ A fugue state is a dissociative state in which the person leaves familiar surroundings, assumes a new identity, and develops amnesia about his previous identity. (It is also described as "flight from himself.") **(PSY)**

▶ Caput succedaneum is edema that develops in and under the fetal scalp during labor and delivery. It resolves spontaneously and presents no danger to the neonate. The edema doesn't cross the suture line. **(MAT)**

▶ Nevus flammeus, or port-wine stain, is a diffuse pink to dark bluish red lesion on the neonate's face or neck. **(MAT)**

▶ Strawberry hemangiomas are raised red birthmarks that may continue to spread up to age 1; complete shrinkage and absorption of hemangiomas may take 7 to 10 years. **(PED)**

▶ Cavernous hemangiomas resemble strawberry hemangiomas but don't disappear with age. **(PED)**

▶ The Guthrie test (a screening test for phenylketonuria) is most reliable if it is done between the second and sixth days after birth and is performed after the neonate has ingested protein. **(MAT)**

▶ To assess coordination of sucking and swallowing, the nurse should observe the neonate's first breast-feeding or sterile water bottle-feeding. **(MAT)**

▶ To establish a milk supply pattern, the mother should breast-feed her infant at least every 4 hours; during the first month, she should breast-feed 8 to 12 times a day (demand feeding). **(MAT)**

▶ The nurse should wear gloves when handling the neonate until after the first bath is given to avoid contact with blood and other body fluids. **(MAT)**

▶ For the infant with a suspected infection, the nurse should maintain isolation and take other appropriate precautions. **(PED)**

▶ If the breast-fed infant is content, has good skin turgor, an adequate number of wet diapers, and normal weight gain, the mother's milk supply is assumed adequate. **(MAT)**

▶ For the female patient of child-bearing age who is undergoing chemotherapy, the nurse should encourage the use of a contraceptive during sexual intercourse because of the risk of fetal damage if she becomes pregnant. **(M-S)**

▶ Pernicious anemia is vitamin B_{12} deficiency caused by a lack of intrinsic factor, which is produced by the gastric mucosal parietal cells. **(M-S)**

▶ To perform pursed-lip breathing, the patient inhales through the nose and exhales slowly and evenly against pursed lips while contracting the abdominal muscles. **(M-S)**

▶ The ascending colostomy drains fluid feces; the descending colostomy drains solid fecal matter. **(FND)**

▶ The patient undergoing chemotherapy should consume a high-calorie, high-protein diet. **(M-S)**

▶ Adverse effects of chemotherapy include bone marrow depression, which causes anemia, leukopenia, and thrombocytopenia; GI epithelial cell irritation, which causes GI ulceration, bleeding, and vomiting; and destruction of hair follicles and skin, which causes alopecia and dermatitis. **(M-S)**

► The infant with celiac disease has fatty, foul-smelling stools. **(PED)**

► The hemoglobin electrophoresis test differentiates between sickle cell trait and sickle cell anemia. **(M-S)**

► A folded towel (called a scrotal bridge) can provide scrotal support for the patient with scrotal edema caused by vasectomy, epididymitis, or orchitis. **(FND)**

► In the supine position, a pregnant patient's enlarged uterus impairs venous return from the lower half of the body to the heart, resulting in supine hypotensive syndrome, also known as inferior vena cava syndrome. **(MAT)**

► Treatment of ankle edema in the pregnant patient consists of frequent rest periods, foot elevation, and avoidance of constricting clothing, such as garters and pantyhose. **(MAT)**

► Erythromycin, clindamycin, and tetracycline produce their antibiotic effects by inhibiting protein synthesis in susceptible organisms. **(M-S)**

► Eruption is the normal presentation of a tooth as it penetrates the gum. **(PED)**

► Recommended weight gain during pregnancy is 25 to 35 lb (11.3 to 15.9 kg). **(MAT)**

► The nurse administers oxygen as prescribed to the patient with heart failure to help overcome hypoxia and dyspnea. **(M-S)**

► Signs and symptoms of small-bowel obstruction include decreased or absent bowel sounds, abdominal distention, decreased flatus, and projectile vomiting. **(M-S)**

► The nurse should use both hands when ventilating a patient with a manual resuscitation bag. (One hand can deliver only 400 cc of air; two hands can deliver 1,000 cc of air.) **(M-S)**

▶ Dosages of methylxanthine agents, such as theophylline (Theo-Dur) and aminophylline (Aminophyllin), should be individualized based on serum drug level, patient response, and adverse reactions. **(M-S)**

▶ When determining which information to give the hospitalized child about a procedure, the nurse should consider the child's developmental — not chronological — age. **(PED)**

▶ The patient should apply a transdermal scopolamine patch (Transderm-Scōp) at least 4 hours before its antiemetic action is needed. **(M-S)**

▶ Early indications of gangrene are edema, pain, redness, tissue darkening, and coldness in the affected body part. **(M-S)**

▶ Ipecac syrup is the emetic of choice because of its effectiveness in evacuating the stomach and relatively low incidence of adverse reactions. **(M-S)**

▶ When giving an injection to the patient with a bleeding disorder, the nurse should use a small-gauge needle and apply pressure to the site for 5 minutes after the injection. **(FND)**

▶ Platelets are the smallest and most fragile formed element of the blood and are essential for coagulation. **(FND)**

▶ To insert a nasogastric tube, the nurse should first instruct the patient to tilt the head back slightly and then insert the tube. When the tube is felt curving at the pharynx, the nurse should tell the patient to tilt the head forward to close the trachea and open the esophagus by swallowing. (Sips of water can facilitate this action.) **(FND)**

▶ Oral iron (ferrous sulfate) may cause green to black stools. **(M-S)**

▶ Polycythemia vera causes pruritus, painful fingers and toes, hyperuricemia, plethora (reddish purple skin and mucosa), weakness, and easy fatigability. **(M-S)**

▶ Rheumatic fever usually is preceded by a group A beta-hemolytic streptococcal infection, such as scarlet fever, otitis

media, streptococcal throat infection, impetigo, or tonsillitis.
(M-S)

▶ A thyroid storm or crisis, an extreme form of hyperthyroidism, is characterized by hyperpyrexia with a temperature of up to 106° F (41.1° C), diarrhea, dehydration, tachycardia up to 200 beats/minute, arrhythmias, extreme irritability, hypotension, and delirium. It may lead to coma, shock, and death.   (M-S)

▶ Tardive dyskinesia, an adverse reaction to long-term antipsychotic drug use, produces involuntary repetitive movements of the tongue, lips, extremities, and trunk.   (M-S)

▶ Tocolytic agents used to treat preterm labor include terbutaline sulfate (Brethine), ritodrine (Yutopar), and magnesium sulfate.
(MAT)

▶ The pregnant woman with hyperemesis gravidarum may require hospitalization to treat dehydration and starvation.   (MAT)

▶ Asthma is bronchoconstriction in response to allergens, such as food, pollen, and drugs; irritants, such as smoke and paint fumes; infections; weather changes; exercise; or gastroesophageal reflux. In the United States, about 5% of children have chronic asthma.   (M-S)

▶ Diaphragmatic hernia is one of the most urgent neonatal surgical emergencies. By compressing and displacing the lungs and heart, this disorder can cause respiratory distress to occur shortly after birth.   (MAT)

▶ Blood cultures help identify the cause of endocarditis; an increased white blood cell count suggests bacterial infection.
(M-S)

▶ Common complications of early pregnancy (up to 20 weeks' gestation) include fetal loss or serious threats to maternal health.   (MAT)

▶ For the patient with an acute aortic dissection, the nursing priority is to maintain the mean arterial pressure between 60 and 65 mm Hg. A vasodilator such as nitroprusside sodium (Nitropress) may be needed to achieve this.   (M-S)

▶ For the patient with heart failure, one of the most important nursing diagnoses is "Decreased cardiac output related to altered myocardial contractility, increased preload and afterload, and altered rate, rhythm, or electrical conduction." **(M-S)**

▶ For the patient receiving peritoneal dialysis, the nurse must monitor body weight and blood urea nitrogen, creatinine, and electrolyte levels. **(M-S)**

▶ Angiotensin-converting enzyme inhibitors, such as captopril (Capoten) and enalapril (Vasotec), decrease blood pressure by interfering with the renin-angiotensin-aldosterone system. **(M-S)**

▶ The patient with stable ventricular tachycardia has a blood pressure and is conscious; therefore, the patient's cardiac output is being maintained, and the nurse must monitor vital signs continuously. **(M-S)**

▶ Angiotensin-converting enzyme inhibitors inhibit the enzyme that converts angiotensin I into angiotensin II, which is a potent vasoconstrictor. Through this action, they reduce peripheral arterial resistance and blood pressure. **(M-S)**

▶ When caring for the patient receiving a diuretic, the nurse should monitor serum electrolyte levels, check vital signs, and observe for orthostatic hypotension. **(M-S)**

▶ According to families whose loved ones are in intensive care units, their four most important needs are to have questions answered honestly, to be assured that the best possible care is being provided, to know the prognosis, and to feel there is hope. **(FND)**

▶ Breast self-examination is one of the most important health habits to teach a female patient and should be done one week after the menstrual period because that is when hormonal effects, which can cause breast lumps and tenderness, are reduced. **(M-S)**

▶ Postmenopausal women should choose a regular time each month to perform breast self-examination (for example, on the day of the month of their birthday). **(M-S)**

▶ The difference between acute and chronic arterial disease is that the acute disease process is life-threatening. **(M-S)**

▶ When preparing the patient for chest tube removal, the nurse should explain that it may cause pain or a burning or pulling sensation. **(M-S)**

▶ Essential hypertensive renal disease usually is characterized by progressive renal impairment. **(M-S)**

▶ Fetal embodiment is a developmental task that occurs in the second trimester, during which the mother may complain that she never gets to sleep because the fetus always gives her a thump when she tries. **(MAT)**

▶ Visualization is a process in which the mother imagines what the child she is carrying is like and becomes acquainted with it. **(MAT)**

▶ Mean arterial pressure (MAP) is calculated using the following formula:

S = systolic pressure   D = diastolic pressure

$$MAP = \frac{(D \times 2) + S}{3}$$

(M-S)

▶ Hemodilution of pregnancy is the increase in blood volume during pregnancy, consisting of plasma and resulting in an imbalance between the ratio of red blood cells to plasma and, therefore, a decrease in hematocrit. **(MAT)**

▶ Mean arterial pressure greater than 100 mm Hg after 20 weeks of pregnancy is considered hypertension. **(MAT)**

▶ Symptoms of supine hypotension syndrome are dizziness, light-headedness, nausea, and vomiting. **(M-S)**

▶ The treatment for supine hypotension syndrome (a condition that sometimes occurs in pregnancy) is to have the patient lie on her left side. **(MAT)**

▶ A contributing factor in dependent edema in the pregnant patient is the increase of femoral venous pressure from 10 mm Hg (normal) to 18 mm Hg (high). **(MAT)**

▶ Hyperpigmentation of the pregnant patient's face, formerly called chloasma and now referred to as melasma, fades after delivery. **(MAT)**

▶ The hormone relaxin, secreted first by the corpus luteum and later by the placenta, relaxes the connective tissue and cartilage of the symphysis pubis and the sacroiliac joint to facilitate passage of the fetus during delivery. **(MAT)**

▶ Progesterone maintains the integrity of the pregnancy by inhibiting uterine motility. **(MAT)**

▶ Ladin's sign, an early indication of pregnancy, is manifested by a softening of a spot on the anterior portion of the uterus just above the uterocervical juncture. **(MAT)**

▶ The abdominal line from the symphysis pubis to the umbilicus changes from linea alba to linea nigra during pregnancy. **(MAT)**

▶ Cold stress in the neonate will affect his circulatory, regulatory, and respiratory systems. **(MAT)**

▶ An immunocompromised patient is at risk for Kaposi sarcoma. **(M-S)**

▶ Further clarification of obstetric data can be achieved by using a system referred to as *F/TPAL:*
F/T: Full-term delivery at 38+ weeks
P: Preterm delivery between 20 and 37 weeks
A: Abortion or loss of fetus before 20 weeks
L: Number of children living (if a child has died, further explanation is needed to clarify the discrepancy in numbers). **(MAT)**

▶ Parity doesn't refer to the number of children delivered, only the number of deliveries. **(MAT)**

▶ Women carrying more than one fetus should be encouraged to gain between 35 and 45 lb (15.9 to 20.4 kg). **(MAT)**

▶ Overweight women should gain between 15 and 25 lb (6.8 and 11.3 kg) during pregnancy. **(MAT)**

▶ The recommended amount of iron supplement for the pregnant patient is 30 to 60 mg daily. **(MAT)**

▶ Drinking six alcoholic beverages a day or a single episode of binge drinking in the first trimester can cause fetal alcohol syndrome. **(MAT)**

▶ Chorionic villus sampling is done at 8 to 12 weeks of pregnancy for early identification of genetic defects. **(MAT)**

▶ Percutaneous umbilical blood sampling is a procedure in which a blood sample is obtained from the umbilical cord to evaluate anemia, genetic defects, and blood incompatibility as well as the need for blood transfusions. **(MAT)**

▶ The period between contractions is referred to as the "interval" or "resting phase." During this phase the uterus and the placenta fill with blood and allow for the exchange of oxygen, carbon dioxide, and nutrients. **(MAT)**

▶ If the patient experiences hypertonic contractions, the uterus doesn't have an opportunity to relax and there is no "interval." As a result, the fetus may experience hypoxia or a rapid delivery. **(MAT)**

▶ Two qualities of myometrium are elasticity, which allows the myometrium to stretch yet maintain tone, and contractility, which allows it to shorten and lengthen in a synchronized pattern. **(MAT)**

▶ Crowning means that the presenting part of the fetus remains visible during the interval between contractions. **(MAT)**

▶ Uterine atony is the failure of the uterus to remain firmly contracted. **(MAT)**

▶ The major cause of uterine atony is a full bladder. **(MAT)**

▶ An infant should be nursed as soon after delivery as possible if the mother wishes to breast-feed. **(MAT)**

▶ A smacking sound, milk dripping from side of the mouth, and sucking noises all indicate improper placement of the infant's mouth over the nipple. **(MAT)**

▶ The infant should be burped before initiating feeding to expel any air in the infant's stomach. **(MAT)**

▶ Most authorities strongly encourage the continuation of breast-feeding both on the affected and unaffected breast of patients with mastitis. **(MAT)**

▶ Expiratory grunting is an abnormal breath sound heard as an infant attempts to breathe out against a closed glottis. **(PED)**

▶ On an infant, the abdomen is the ideal place to check skin turgor. **(PED)**

▶ Normal urine output for an infant is 1 to 3 ml/kg of body weight per hour. **(PED)**

▶ The lag between head movement and eye movement is referred to as "doll's eye movement" and is normal. **(M-S)**

▶ Neonates are nearsighted and focus on items held 10″ to 12″ (25.4 to 30.5 cm) away. **(MAT)**

▶ Low-set ears in a neonate are associated with chromosomal abnormalities such as Down syndrome. **(MAT)**

▶ Meconium is usually passed in the first 24 hours; however, it may take up to 72 hours. **(MAT)**

▶ Breast-fed infants tend to pass stools that are looser and pastier than those of bottle-fed babies. **(PED)**

▶ Male infants born with hypospadias shouldn't be circumcised at birth because the foreskin may be needed for constructive surgery. **(MAT)**

▶ Circumcision carried out by a rabbi is called a "bris." **(PED)**

▶ The most desirable diet for an infant up to age 6 months is breast milk. **(PED)**

▶ An infant is ready for the addition of solids to his diet when he meets these indicators: 1) has doubled his weight, 2) demands between 8 and 10 feedings in a 24-hour period, 3) drinks in excess of a quart of formula a day, and 4) always seems hungry. **(PED)**

▶ Solids are introduced to the infant in the following order: rice cereal, fruits, oatmeal, vegetables, and meat. **(PED)**

▶ The normal blood level of glucose in the neonate is 45 to 90 mg/dl. **(MAT)**

▶ Hepatitis B vaccine is usually given within 48 hours of birth. **(MAT)**

▶ Hepatitis B immune globulin is usually given within 12 hours of birth. **(MAT)**

▶ HELLP syndrome is an unusual variation of pregnancy-induced hypertension. The acronym stands for hemolysis, elevated liver enzymes, and low platelets. **(MAT)**

▶ Maternal serum alpha-fetoprotein is detectable at 7 weeks and peaks in the third trimester. High levels detected between the 16th and 18th week are associated with neural tube defects, and low levels are associated with Down syndrome. **(MAT)**

▶ An arrest of descent occurs when the fetus fails to descend through the pelvic cavity during labor and is often associated with cephalopelvic disproportion. Cesarean intervention may be required. **(MAT)**

▶ A late sign of preeclampsia is epigastric pain secondary to severe edema of the liver. **(MAT)**

▶ After delivery, blood pressure returns to normal during the puerperal period in the patient with preeclampsia. **(MAT)**

▶ Third spacing of fluid is a shifting of fluid from the intravascular space to the interstitial space, where it remains. **(M-S)**

▶ Chronic pain is described as any pain that lasts longer than 6 months; acute pain lasts less than 6 months. **(M-S)**

▶ A double-bind communication exists when the verbal message contradicts the nonverbal message and the receiver is unsure of which message to respond to. **(FND)**

▶ A nonjudgmental attitude displayed by the nurse demonstrates that she neither approves nor disapproves of the patient. **(FND)**

▶ In a psychiatric setting, the patient should be able to predict the nurse's behavior and expect consistent positive attitudes and approaches. **(PSY)**

▶ When establishing a schedule for a one-to-one interaction with the patient, the nurse should state how long the conversation will last and strictly adhere to the time limit. **(PSY)**

▶ Target symptoms are those that the patient and others find most distressing. **(FND)**

▶ The mechanism of action of a phenothiazine derivative is to block dopamine receptors in the brain. **(M-S)**

▶ Thought broadcasting is a type of delusion in which the person believes that his thoughts are being broadcast for the world to hear. **(PSY)**

▶ Advise the patient to take aspirin on an empty stomach with a full glass of water and to avoid foods with acid such as coffee, citrus fruits, and cola. **(FND)**

▶ Advise the patient not to take bisacodyl, antacids, and dairy products all at the same time. **(M-S)**

▶ Advise the patient on digoxin to avoid foods high in fiber, such as bran cereal and prunes. **(M-S)**

▶ The patient on diuretics should avoid foods with monosodium glutamate as it can cause a tightening of chest and flushing of face. **(M-S)**

▶ Furosemide (Lasix) should be taken 1 hour before meals. **(M-S)**

▶ Advise the patient on griseofulvin (Grisovin FP) to maintain a high-fat diet, which enhances the secretion of bile. **(M-S)**

▶ Advise the patient to take oral iron products with citrus drinks to enhance absorption. **(M-S)**

▶ Isoniazid should be taken on an empty stomach with a full glass of water. **(M-S)**

▶ Foods high in protein decrease the absorption of levodopa. **(M-S)**

▶ Lithium carbonate should be taken with foods and the patient shouldn't restrict his sodium intake. **(PSY)**

▶ The patient on lithium carbonate should stop the medication and call the doctor if he experiences vomiting, drowsiness, or muscle weakness. **(PSY)**

▶ The patient taking tetracycline shouldn't take iron supplements or antacids. **(M-S)**

▶ The patient on warfarin (Coumadin) should avoid foods high in vitamin K, such as liver and green leafy vegetables. **(M-S)**

▶ Cottage cheese, cream cheese, yogurt, and sour cream are permitted in the diet of the patient taking a monoamine oxidase inhibitor for depression. **(PSY)**

▶ The normal value for cholesterol is less than 200 mg/dl. (The normal value for low-density lipoproteins is 60 to180 mg/dl and high-density lipoproteins is 30 to 80 mg/dl). **(M-S)**

▶ The normal cardiac output for the 155-lb (70-kg) adult is 5 to 6 L/minute. **(M-S)**

▶ A pulmonary artery pressure catheter (Swan-Ganz) measures the pressure in the cardiac chambers. **(M-S)**

▶ Severe chest pain aggravated by breathing and described as "sharp," "stabbing," or "knifelike" is consistent with pericarditis. **(M-S)**

▶ A pulse that is loud and bounding and that rapidly rises and falls is described as water-hammer pulse and can be caused by emotional excitement and aortic insufficiency. **(M-S)**

▶ A pathologic splitting of S_2 is normally heard between inspiration and expiration and occurs in right bundle-branch block.
(M-S)

▶ Pink frothy sputum is associated with pulmonary edema; frank hemoptysis may be associated with pulmonary embolism.
(M-S)

▶ An aortic aneurysm can be heard just over the umbilical area and can be detected as an abdominal pulsation (bruit). **(M-S)**

▶ In grading heart murmurs, grade 1 is faint and heard after the examiner "tunes in"; grade 2 is heard immediately; grade 3 is moderately loud; grade 4 is loud; grade 5 is very loud but only heard with a stethoscope; and grade 6 is very loud and heard without a stethoscope. **(M-S)**

▶ Clot formation during cardiac catheterization is minimized by the administration of 4,000 to 5,000 units of heparin. **(M-S)**

▶ Most complications that arise from cardiac catheterization are associated with the puncture site. **(M-S)**

▶ Allergic symptoms associated with iodine-based contrast media used in cardiac catheterization include urticaria, nausea and vomiting, and flushing. **(M-S)**

▶ To ensure that blood flow hasn't been compromised, the nurse should mark the peripheral pulses distal to the cutdown site to aid in locating the pulses following the procedure. **(M-S)**

▶ The extremity used for the cutdown site should remain straight for 4 to 6 hours. If an antecubital vessel was used, use an armboard. If a femoral artery was used, keep the patient on bed rest for 6 to 12 hours. **(M-S)**

▶ The doctor should be notified immediately if the patient experiences numbness or tingling in the extremity after a cutdown.
(M-S)

▶ Following cardiac catheterization, encourage fluid intake to aid in flushing the contrast medium through the kidneys. **(M-S)**

▶ Risks to the patient undergoing a pulmonary artery catheterization are pulmonary artery infarction, pulmonary embolism, injury to the heart valves, and injury to the myocardium. **(M-S)**

▶ Pulmonary artery wedge pressure is a direct indicator of left ventricular pressure. **(M-S)**

▶ Pulmonary artery wedge pressure greater than 18 to 20 mm Hg indicates increased left ventricular pressure, as seen in left ventricular failure. **(M-S)**

▶ When taking a pulmonary artery wedge pressure reading, place the patient in a supine position with the head of the bed elevated no more than 25 degrees. **(M-S)**

▶ Pulmonary artery pressure, which indicates right and left ventricular pressure, is taken with the balloon deflated. **(M-S)**

▶ Pulmonary artery systolic pressure indicates the peak pressure generated by the right ventricle. Pulmonary artery diastolic pressure indicates the lowest pressure in the pulmonary artery. **(M-S)**

▶ The normal adult pulmonary artery systolic pressure is 15 to 25 mm Hg. **(M-S)**

▶ The normal adult pulmonary artery diastolic pressure is 8 to 12 mm Hg. **(M-S)**

▶ The normal oxygen saturation of venous blood is 75%. **(M-S)**

▶ Central venous pressure is the amount of pressure in the superior vena cava and the right atrium. **(M-S)**

▶ The normal central venous pressure is 2 to 8 mm Hg or 3 to 10 cm H_2O. **(M-S)**

▶ A decrease in central venous pressure indicates a fall in circulating fluid volume as seen in shock. **(M-S)**

▶ A rise in central venous pressure is associated with an increase in circulating volume as seen in renal failure. **(M-S)**

▶ If a central venous pressure reading is to be obtained when the patient is on a ventilator, the reading should be taken at the end of the expiratory cycle. **(M-S)**

▶ To ensure an accurate baseline central venous pressure reading, the zero point of the transducer must be at the level of the right atrium. **(M-S)**

▶ A blood pressure reading obtained via intra-arterial pressure monitoring may be 10 mm Hg higher than one obtained using a blood pressure cuff. **(M-S)**

▶ Mönckeberg's sclerosis is a condition in which calcium deposits form in the medial layer of the arterial walls. **(M-S)**

▶ The symptoms associated with coronary artery disease usually don't appear until plaque has narrowed the vessels by at least 75%. **(M-S)**

▶ Symptoms of coronary artery disease will only appear when there is an imbalance between the demand for oxygenated blood and its availability. **(M-S)**

▶ Percutaneous transluminal coronary angioplasty is an invasive procedure in which a balloon-tipped catheter is inserted into a blocked artery and inflated to compress plaque against the intimal layer of the artery to open it. **(M-S)**

▶ Before a percutaneous transluminal coronary angioplasty, an anticoagulant (such as aspirin) is usually administered to the patient; during the procedure he's given heparin, a calcium agonist, or nitroglycerin to reduce the risk of coronary artery spasms. **(M-S)**

▶ A coronary artery bypass graft is a surgical procedure to bypass a blocked coronary artery by using the saphenous vein from a thigh or lower leg. **(M-S)**

▶ When a vein is used to bypass an artery, the vein is reversed so that the valves don't interfere with blood flow. **(M-S)**

▶ During a coronary artery bypass graft, the patient's heart is stopped to sew the new vessel in place. Blood flow to the body is maintained by a cardiopulmonary bypass. **(M-S)**

▶ During an anginal attack, the cells of the heart convert to anaerobic metabolism, which leaves lactic acid as a waste product. As the level of lactic acid increases, pain develops. **(M-S)**

▶ Pain that is described as "sharp" or "knifelike" is not consistent with angina pectoris. **(M-S)**

▶ Anginal pain typically lasts for 5 minutes; however, attacks associated with heavy meals or extreme emotional distress may last 15 to 20 minutes. **(M-S)**

▶ "Exertion-pain-rest-relief" is consistent with stable angina. **(M-S)**

▶ Unstable angina, unlike stable angina, can occur without exertion and is considered a precursor to a myocardial infarction. **(M-S)**

▶ If the patient is scheduled for a stress electrocardiogram, he should notify the staff if he has taken nitrates. (If he has, the test needs to be rescheduled.) **(M-S)**

▶ An exercise mechanism, such as a treadmill or exercise bike, is used for a stress electrocardiogram. Activity is increased until the patient reaches 85% of his maximum heart rate. **(M-S)**

▶ Patients taking nitroglycerin for a long time often develop a tolerance, which reduces the effectiveness of nitrates. Therefore, a 12-hour drug-free period is usually used at night. **(M-S)**

▶ Beta blockers such as propranolol (Inderal) reduce the workload on the heart, thereby decreasing the oxygen demand, and also slow the heart rate. **(M-S)**

▶ Calcium channel blockers include nifedipine (Procardia), which is used to treat angina; verapamil (Calan, Isoptin), which is used primarily as a antiarrhythmic; and diltiazem (Cardizem), which combines the effects of nifedipine and verapamil without the adverse effects. **(M-S)**

▶ The posthospitalized myocardial patient should avoid heavy meals, smoking, coffee, extremes in temperatures and weather, and strenuous exercises. **(M-S)**

▶ The patient who is experiencing anginal pain that radiates or worsens and doesn't subside should be seen at an emergency medical facility. **(M-S)**

▶ Cardiac cells can withstand 20 minutes of ischemia before cell death occurs. **(M-S)**

▶ The most common site of injury during a myocardial infarction is the anterior wall of the left ventricle near the apex. **(M-S)**

▶ The infarcted tissue of a myocardial infarction causes significant Q-wave changes on an electrocardiogram that remain evident even after the myocardium heals. **(M-S)**

▶ CK-MB, an isoenzyme specific to the heart, increases 4 to 6 hours after a myocardial infarction and peaks at 12 to 18 hours. It returns to normal in 3 to 4 days. **(M-S)**

▶ Patients who survive a myocardial infarction and have no other cardiovascular pathology usually require 6 to 12 weeks for a full recovery. **(M-S)**

▶ Fifty percent of patients who survive a myocardial infarction (MI) will die of an MI within 5 years; 75% will die within 10 years of a massive MI. **(M-S)**

▶ Following a myocardial infarction, the patient is at the greatest risk for sudden death during the first 24 hours. **(M-S)**

▶ Following a myocardial infarction, the crucial period for salvaging the myocardium is considered to be the first 6 hours. **(M-S)**

▶ Following a myocardial infarction, the doctor should be notified if the patient is experiencing more than three premature ventricular contractions per minute. **(M-S)**

▶ Following a myocardial infarction, increasing vascular resistance through the use of vasopressors, such as dopamine and levarterenol, can raise blood pressure. **(M-S)**

▶ Clinical manifestations of heart failure include distended neck veins, weight gain, orthopnea, crackles, and enlarged liver. **(M-S)**

▶ Risk factors associated with embolism are increased blood viscosity, decreased circulation, prolonged bed rest, and increased blood coagulability. **(M-S)**

▶ Antiembolism stockings should be worn around the clock except twice a day for 30 minutes when they are removed for skin care. **(M-S)**

▶ Before the nurse puts antiembolism stockings back on the patient, the patient should lie with his feet elevated 6" (15 cm) for 20 minutes. **(M-S)**

▶ Dressler's syndrome is termed "late pericarditis" because it occurs approximately 6 weeks to 6 months after a myocardial infarction and is manifested by pericardial pain and a fever that lasts longer than 1 week. **(M-S)**

▶ In phase I following a myocardial infarction, the patient is kept on a clear liquid diet and bed rest with the use of a bedside commode for the first 24 hours. **(M-S)**

▶ In phase I following a myocardial infarction, the patient is up and out of bed for 15 to 20 minutes in a chair on the second day. The number of times the patient goes to the chair and the length of time in the chair are increased depending on endurance. In phase II, the length of time out of bed and the distance to the chair are increased. **(M-S)**

▶ After transfer from the cardiac care unit, the post–myocardial infarction patient is allowed to walk the halls as his endurance increases. **(M-S)**

▶ Sexual intercourse with a known partner can usually be resumed 4 to 8 weeks after a myocardial infarction. **(M-S)**

▶ A cardiac-care patient should avoid eating or drinking alcoholic beverages before engaging in sexual intercourse. **(M-S)**

▶ The ambulation goal for a post-myocardial infarction patient is 2 miles in 60 minutes. **(M-S)**

▶ A post-myocardial infarction patient who doesn't have a strenuous job may be able to return to work full-time in 8 or 9 weeks. **(M-S)**

▶ Stroke volume is the amount of blood ejected from the heart with each heartbeat. **(M-S)**

▶ The force that the ventricle must develop during systole to eject the stroke volume is termed afterload. **(M-S)**

▶ The three-point position (patient upright and leaning forward with hands on knees) is characteristic of orthopnea as seen in left-side heart failure. **(M-S)**

▶ Paroxysmal nocturnal dyspnea indicates a severe form of pulmonary congestion in which the patient awakens in the middle of the night with a feeling of being suffocated. **(M-S)**

▶ Clinical manifestations of pulmonary edema include breathlessness, nasal flaring, use of accessory muscles to breath, and frothy sputum. **(M-S)**

▶ A late sign of heart failure is a decrease in cardiac output, causing blood flow to the kidneys to decrease, resulting in oliguria. **(M-S)**

▶ A late sign of heart failure is anasarca (generalized edema). **(M-S)**

▶ Dependent edema is an early sign of right-sided heart failure and is seen in the legs where increased capillary hydrostatic pressure overwhelms plasma protein causing a shift of fluid from the capillary beds to the interstitial spaces. **(M-S)**

▶ Dependent edema, most noticeable at the end of the day, usually starts in the feet and ankles and continues upward. **(M-S)**

▶ For the recumbent patient, edema is usually seen in the presacral area. **(M-S)**

▶ Signs of urinary tract infection include frequency, urgency, and dysuria. **(M-S)**

▶ Tertiary-intention healing is a process in which the closure of the wound is delayed when a wound is infected or there is considerable edema. **(M-S)**

▶ The patient who has had supratentorial surgery should have the head of the bed elevated to 30 degrees. **(M-S)**

▶ An acid-ash diet acidifies the urine. **(M-S)**

▶ Vitamin C and cranberry juice acidify urine. **(M-S)**

▶ The patient taking probenecid (ColBENEMID) for gout should be instructed to take the medication with food. **(M-S)**

▶ If wound dehiscence is suspected, tell the patient to lie down and then examine the wound and monitor his vital signs. Any abnormal findings should be reported to the doctor. **(M-S)**

▶ Miotics, such as pilocarpine, are administered to the patient with acute glaucoma to increase the outflow of aqueous humor. **(M-S)**

▶ Zoster immune globulin is administered to the patient to stimulate immunity to varicella. **(M-S)**

▶ The most common symptoms associated with compartmental syndrome are pain not relieved by analgesics, loss of movement, loss of sensation, pain with passive movement, and lack of pulse. **(M-S)**

▶ To help the patient with multiple sclerosis relieve muscle spasms, administer baclofen (Lioresal) as ordered, give a warm soothing bath, and teach progressive relaxation techniques. **(M-S)**

▶ The patient with a cervical injury and impairment at C5 should be able to lift shoulders and elbows partially but would have no sensation below the clavicle. **(M-S)**

▶ The patient with cervical injury and impairment at C6 should be able to lift shoulders, elbows, and wrists partially but would have no sensation below the clavicle except a little in the arms and thumb. **(M-S)**

▶ The patient with cervical injury and impairment at C7 should be able to lift shoulders, elbows, wrists, and hands partially but would have no sensation below the midchest. **(M-S)**

▶ Injuries to the spinal cord at C3 and above may be fatal because of a loss of innervation to the diaphragm and intercostal muscles. **(M-S)**

▶ For every patient problem, there is a nursing diagnosis; for every nursing diagnosis, there is a goal; and for every goal, there are interventions designed to make the goal a reality. The keys to answering examination questions correctly are identifying the problem presented, formulating a goal for that specific problem, and then selecting the intervention from the choices provided that will enable the patient to reach that goal. **(FND)**

▶ Signs of meningeal irritation seen in meningitis include nuchal rigidity, a positive Brudzinski's sign, and a positive Kernig's sign. **(M-S)**

▶ Laboratory values indicating pneumomeningitis include elevated cerebrospinal fluid protein (over 100 mg/dl), decreased cerebrospinal fluid glucose (40 mg/dl), and increased white blood cell count. **(M-S)**

▶ The first nursing action to promote rest in the very young child in a hospital setting is to decrease environmental stimulation. **(PED)**

▶ To promote sleep in a very young child in a hospital setting, the nurse should ask the parents about the child's sleep rituals. **(PED)**

▶ Before undergoing magnetic resonance imaging, the patient should remove all objects containing metal, such as watches, bras, and jewelry. **(M-S)**

▶ Usually food and medicine aren't restricted before magnetic resonance imaging. **(M-S)**

▶ Patients undergoing magnetic resonance imaging should know that they can ask questions during the procedure; however, they may be asked to lie still at certain times.   **(M-S)**

▶ If a contrast medium is used during magnetic resonance imaging, advise the patient that he may experience diuresis as the medium is flushed from the body.   **(M-S)**

▶ The Tzanck test is used to confirm herpes genitalis.   **(M-S)**

▶ Hepatitis C is spread primarily through blood (posttransfusion or persons working with blood products), personal contact and, possibly, the fecal-oral route.   **(M-S)**

▶ The best soak for an open, infected, draining wound is a hot-moist dressing.   **(M-S)**

▶ A sputum culture is the confirmation test for tuberculosis.   **(M-S)**

▶ Dexamethasone (Decadron) is a steroidal anti-inflammatory used in the treatment of adrenal insufficiency.   **(M-S)**

▶ Signs of increased intracranial pressure include alteration in level of consciousness, restlessness, irritability, and pupillary changes.   **(M-S)**

▶ The patient with a lower limb amputation should be instructed to assume a prone position at least twice a day.   **(M-S)**

▶ During the first 24 hours following amputation, the residual limb is elevated on a pillow. After that time, the limb is placed flat to reduce the risk of hip flexion contractures.   **(M-S)**

▶ A tourniquet should be in full view at the bedside of the patient with an amputation.   **(M-S)**

▶ An emergency tracheostomy set should be kept at the bedside of the patient suspected of having epiglottitis.   **(M-S)**

▶ Rocky Mountain spotted fever is spread through the bite of a tick harboring the *Rickettsia* organism.   **(M-S)**

▶ The key word to use in reporting suspected cases of child abuse to the appropriate authorities is is "suspected." **(PED)**

▶ The patient with acquired immunodeficiency syndrome shouldn't share razors or toothbrushes with others; however, there are no special precautions regarding dinnerware or laundry services. **(M-S)**

▶ Because antifungal creams may stain clothing, patients should be advised to use sanitary napkins. **(M-S)**

▶ Antifungal creams should be inserted high in the vagina at bedtime. **(M-S)**

▶ The patient experiencing a seizure usually requires protection from the environment only; however, anyone needing airway management should be turned on his side. **(M-S)**

▶ Status epilepticus is treated with I.V. diphenylhydantoin. **(M-S)**

▶ A skin graft from an animal is termed a xenograft. **(M-S)**

▶ Fidelity means loyalty and can be shown as a commitment to the profession of nursing and to the patient. **(FND)**

▶ Giving an I.M. injection against the patient's will and without legal authority is battery. **(FND)**

▶ An example of a third-party payor is an insurance company. **(FND)**

▶ The formula for calculating the drops per minute for an I.V. infusion is as follows:

$$\frac{(\text{volume to be infused} \times \text{drip factor})}{\text{time in minutes}} = \text{drops/minute}$$

(FND)

▶ On-call medication should be given within 5 minutes of receipt of the call. **(FND)**

▶ Generally, the best method to determine the cultural or spiritual needs of the patient is to ask him. **(FND)**

▶ An incident report shouldn't be made part of a patient's record but is an in-house document for the purpose of correcting the problem. **(FND)**

▶ Critical pathways are a multidisciplinary guideline for patient care. **(FND)**

▶ The antidote for magnesium sulfate is calcium gluconate 10%. **(M-S)**

▶ Allergic reactions to a blood transfusion are flushing, wheezing, urticaria, and rash. **(M-S)**

▶ The child with asthma can promote expansion of the lungs by blowing a pinwheel. **(PED)**

▶ The patient with a history of basal cell carcinoma should avoid sun exposure. **(M-S)**

▶ When potent, nitroglycerin causes a slight stinging sensation under the tongue. **(M-S)**

▶ For an estriol level, urine is collected for 24 hours. **(MAT)**

▶ An estriol level is used to assess fetal well-being, maternal renal functioning, and a pregnancy complicated by diabetes. **(MAT)**

▶ Water accumulating in a ventilator tube should be removed. **(M-S)**

▶ When the patient appears to be "fighting a ventilator," the patient is holding his breath or breathing out on an inspiratory cycle. **(M-S)**

▶ An antineoplastic drug used in the treatment of breast cancer is tamoxifen (Nolvadex). **(M-S)**

▶ Adverse effects of vincristine (Oncovin) are alopecia, nausea, and vomiting. **(M-S)**

▶ The pregnant patient with vaginal bleeding shouldn't have a pelvic examination. **(MAT)**

▶ An indication that a hypertensive crisis is normalizing is increased urine output. **(M-S)**

▶ If the patient receiving I.V. chemotherapy drugs complains of pain at the insertion site, the nurse should stop the I.V. infusion immediately. **(M-S)**

▶ Extravasation is the leakage of fluid into surrounding tissue from a vein being used for I.V. therapy. **(M-S)**

▶ Clinical signs of prostate cancer are dribbling, hesitancy, and decreased urinary force. **(M-S)**

▶ Digitalis glycosides increase cardiac contractility. **(M-S)**

▶ Adverse effects of digitalis glycosides include headache, hypotension, nausea and vomiting, and yellow-green halos around lights. **(M-S)**

▶ A T tube should be clamped during meal hour to aid in fat digestion. **(M-S)**

▶ A T tube usually remains in place for 10 days. **(M-S)**

▶ During a vertigo attack, the patient with Ménière's disease should be instructed to lie down on his side with his eyes closed. **(M-S)**

▶ When prioritizing nursing diagnoses, use this hierarchy: (1) problems associated with airway, (2) those concerning breathing, and (3) those related to circulation. **(FND)**

▶ The two nursing diagnoses with the highest priority that the nurse can assign are *Ineffective airway clearance* and *Ineffective breathing pattern*. **(FND)**

▶ When maintaining a Jackson-Pratt drainage system, the nurse should squeeze the reservoir and expel the air before recapping. **(M-S)**

▶ Sensory overload is a state in which sensory stimulation exceeds one's capacity to tolerate or process it. **(PSY)**

▶ Symptoms of sensory overload include a feeling of distress and hyperarousal with impaired thinking and concentration. **(PSY)**

▶ Sensory deprivation is a state in which the overall sensory input is decreased. **(PSY)**

▶ A sign of sensory deprivation includes an increase in stimulation from the environment or from within oneself, such as daydreaming, inactivity, sleeping excessively, and reminiscing. **(PSY)**

▶ A subjective sign that a sitz bath has been effective is the patient expresses a decrease in pain or discomfort. **(FND)**

▶ For the nursing diagnosis *Diversional activity deficit* to be valid, the patient must make the statement that he's "bored, there is nothing to do" or words to that effect. **(FND)**

▶ The most appropriate nursing diagnosis for an individual who doesn't speak English is *Communication, impaired, related to inability to speak dominant language (English).* **(FND)**

▶ The family of the patient who has been diagnosed as hearing impaired should be instructed to face the individual when they speak to him. **(FND)**

▶ The most common symptom associated with sleep apnea is snoring. **(M-S)**

▶ Up to age 3, the pinna should be pulled down and back to straighten the eustachian tube before instilling medication. **(FND)**

▶ When administering eyedrops, the nurse should waste the first drop and instill the medication in the lower conjunctival sac to prevent injury to the cornea. **(FND)**

▶ When administering eye ointment, the nurse should waste the first bead of medication and then apply the medication from the inner to the outer canthus. **(FND)**

▶ Histamine is released during an inflammatory response. **(M-S)**

▶ In dealing with a patient who has a severe speech impediment, the nurse should minimize background noise and not interrupt the patient when he attempts to speak. **(M-S)**

▶ Fever and night sweats, hallmark signs of tuberculosis, may not be present in elderly patients with the disease. **(M-S)**

▶ A suitable dressing for wound debridement is wet-to-dry. **(M-S)**

▶ Drinking warm milk at bedtime aids sleeping because of the natural sedative effect of the amino acid tryptophan. **(M-S)**

▶ The three stages of general adaptation syndrome are alarm, resistance, and exhaustion. **(PSY)**

▶ The initial step in promoting sleep in a hospitalized patient is to minimize environmental stimulation. **(M-S)**

▶ Before moving the patient, assess how much exertion the patient is permitted, the patient's physical ability, and his ability to understand instruction as well as one's own strength and ability to move the patient. **(M-S)**

▶ The patient in a restraint should be checked every 30 minutes and the restraint loosened every 2 hours to permit range of motion of the extremities. **(M-S)**

▶ Antibiotics that are to be given four times a day should be given at 6 a.m., 12 p.m., 6 p.m., and 12 a.m. to minimize disruption of sleep. **(M-S)**

▶ When removing gloves and mask, the gloves, which most likely contain pathogens and are soiled, should be removed first. **(FND)**

▶ Sundowner syndrome is observed in patients who become more confused toward the evening. To counter this, the nurse should turn a light on. **(M-S)**

▶ Crutches should placed 6″ (15 cm) in front of the patient and 6″ to the side to assume a tripod position. **(FND)**

▶ The primary goal for the patient who has somnambulism is to prevent injury by providing a safe environment. **(M-S)**

▶ Naloxone (Narcan) should be kept at the bedside of the patient who is receiving patient-controlled analgesia. **(M-S)**

▶ Listening is the most effective communication technique. **(FND)**

▶ Hypnotic medications decrease rapid eye movement sleep but increase the overall amount of sleep. **(M-S)**

▶ Before teaching any procedure to the patient, the nurse must first assess the patient's willingness to learn and his current knowledge. **(FND)**

▶ A sudden wave of overwhelming sleepiness is a symptom of narcolepsy. **(M-S)**

▶ Process recording is a method of evaluating one's communication effectiveness. **(FND)**

▶ When feeding the elderly, limit high-carbohydrate foods because of the risk of glucose intolerance. **(FND)**

▶ When feeding the elderly, feed essential foods first. **(FND)**

▶ Passive range of motion maintains joint mobility whereas resistive exercises increase muscle mass. **(FND)**

▶ Isometric exercises are performed on an extremity in a cast. **(FND)**

▶ The diabetic patient should be instructed to buy shoes in the afternoon because feet are usually the largest at that time of the day. **(M-S)**

▶ A maladaptive response to stress is drinking alcohol or smoking excessively. **(PSY)**

▶ A back rub is an example of the gate-control theory of pain. **(FND)**

▶ Anything below the waist is considered unsterile, a sterile field becomes unsterile when it comes in contact with any unsterile item, a sterile field must be continuously monitored, and the 1″ (2.5 cm) border around a sterile field is considered unsterile. **(FND)**

▶ A "shift to the left" is evident when there is an increase in immature cells (bands) in the blood to fight an infection. **(FND)**

▶ A "shift to the right" is evident when there is an increase in mature cells in the blood as seen in advanced liver diseases and pernicious anemia. **(FND)**

▶ If surgery is scheduled late in the afternoon, the surgeon may approve a light breakfast. **(M-S)**

▶ A hearing aid is usually left in place during surgery for communicating with the patient. The operating room team should be notified of its presence. **(M-S)**

▶ Before administering preoperative medication, make sure that an informed consent form has been signed and attached to the patient's record. **(FND)**

▶ The nurse should monitor the patient for central nervous system depression for 24 hours after receiving nitrous oxide. **(M-S)**

▶ Proper position of the adult in a postanesthesia care unit is head to the side and chin extended upward. The Sims' position can also be used unless contraindicated. **(M-S)**

▶ The first action upon admission to a postanesthesia care unit is to assess airway patency of the patient. **(M-S)**

▶ If the patient is admitted to the postanesthesia care unit without pharyngeal reflex, he is positioned on his side and the nurse stays at the bedside until the gag reflex returns. **(M-S)**

▶ In a postanesthesia care unit, vital signs are routinely taken every 15 minutes, or more often if indicated, until the patient is stable. **(M-S)**

▶ The T tube in a postanesthesia care unit should be unclamped and attached to a drainage system. **(M-S)**

▶ After the patient receives anesthesia, the nurse needs to observe the patient for a drop in blood pressure or evidence of labored breathing. **(M-S)**

► If during the postanesthesia assessment, the patient starts going into shock, the nurse should administer oxygen to the patient, place him in a Trendelenburg position, and increase the I.V. fluid rate per the doctor's order or the policy of the postanesthesia care unit.   **(M-S)**

► Types of benign tumors include myxomas, fibromas, lipomas, osteomas, and chondroma.   **(M-S)**

► Malignant tumors include sarcoma, basal cell carcinoma, fibrosarcoma, osteosarcoma, myxosarcoma, chondrosarcoma, and adenocarcinoma.   **(M-S)**

► Palliative surgery for the cancer patient is performed to reduce pain, relieve airway obstruction, relieve GI obstruction, prevent hemorrhage, relieve pressure on the brain and spinal cord, drain abscesses, and remove or drain infected tumors.   **(M-S)**

► The patient undergoing radiation implant therapy should be kept in a private room to reduce the risk of exposure to others, including nursing personnel.   **(M-S)**

► The nurse should spend no more than 30 minutes per 8-hour shift in providing care to the patient with a radiation implant.   **(FND)**

► The nurse should stand near the patient's shoulders for cervical implants and at the foot of the bed for head and neck implants.   **(FND)**

► The nurse should never be assigned to care for more than one patient with radiation implants.   **(FND)**

► Long-handled forceps and a lead-lined container should be in the room of the patient who has a radiation implant.   **(FND)**

► Generally, patients who have the same infection and are in strict isolation can share the same room.   **(FND)**

► Diseases requiring strict isolation include chickenpox, diphtheria, and viral hemorrhagic fever such as Marburg virus disease.   **(FND)**

▶ In total knee replacement surgery, keep the knee in maximum extension for 3 days. **(M-S)**

▶ Partial weight bearing is allowed approximately 1 week after total knee replacement and weight bearing to the point of pain is allowed at 2 weeks. **(M-S)**

▶ Sjögren's syndrome is a chronic inflammatory disorder associated with a decrease in salivation and lacrimation. Clinical manifestations include a dry mouth, dry eyes, and a dry vagina. **(M-S)**

▶ When treating a child with bacterial meningitis, I.V. antibiotic therapy is used so that the medication will penetrate the blood-brain barrier. **(PED)**

▶ Normal values of cerebrospinal fluid include protein 15 to 45 mg/100 ml, glucose (fasting) 50 to 80 mg/100 ml, red blood cells 0, white blood cells 0 to 5/µl, pH 7.3, and potassium ions 2.9 mmol/L. **(M-S)**

▶ In identifying whether a cranial nerve is a motor nerve, use the following pneumonic:

I,   II, III,   IV,   V, VI, VII,   VIII, IX, X,   XI,   XII
Some **S**ay **M**arry **M**oney, **B**ut **M**y **B**rother **S**ays **B**ad **B**usiness **M**arry **M**oney.

Here's how to interpret the pneumonic: If the word begins with an S, it is a sensory nerve; if it starts with an M, it is a motor nerve; and if it starts with a B, it is both a sensory and motor nerve. **(M-S)**

▶ The Glasgow Coma Scale evaluates level of consciousness, pupil reaction, and motor activity; a score between 3 and 15 is possible. **(M-S)**

▶ When assessing the patient's pupils, the nurse should keep in mind that anisocoria, unequal pupils of 1 mm or larger, is found in approximately 17% of the population. **(M-S)**

▶ Homonymous hemianopia is a condition of defective vision in which the patient sees only half of the visual field with each eye; thus, the patient sees only half of normal vision. **(M-S)**

▶ Passive range-of-motion exercises are usually started 24 hours after a cerebrovascular accident and are performed four times a day. **(M-S)**

▶ The medical management goal in treating the patient with a transient ischemic attack is to prevent a cerebrovascular accident, and in this effort the patient is administered antihypertensive drugs, antiplatelet drugs or aspirin, and in some cases warfarin (Coumadin). **(M-S)**

▶ The patient with an intraperitoneal shunt should be observed for increased abdominal girth. **(M-S)**

▶ Digestion of carbohydrates begins in the mouth. **(M-S)**

▶ Digestion of fats begins in the stomach but is done predominantly in the small intestine. **(M-S)**

▶ Dietary sources of magnesium are fish, grains, and nuts. **(M-S)**

▶ A rough estimate of serum osmolarity is twice the value of serum sodium. **(M-S)**

▶ In determining acid-base problems, first note the pH. If it's above 7.45, it's a problem of alkalosis; if it's below 7.35, it's a problem of acidosis. Next look at the partial pressure of arterial carbon dioxide ($Paco_2$). This is the respiratory indicator. If the pH indicates acidosis and the $Paco_2$ indicates acidosis (above 45 mm Hg), then there is a match and the source of the problem is respiration and is referred to as respiratory acidosis. If the pH indicates alkalosis and the $Paco_2$ also indicates alkalosis (below 35 mm Hg), then there is a match and the source of the problem is respiration and is referred to as respiratory alkalosis. If the $Paco_2$ is normal, then look at the bicarbonate (HCO_3^-), which is the metabolic indicator, and note whether it's acidic (less than 22 mEq/L) or alkaline (greater than 26 mEq/L). Determine which value the pH matches; it will determine whether it's metabolic acidosis or metabolic alkalosis. If both the $Paco_2$ and HCO_3^- are abnormal, then the body is compensating. If the pH has returned to normal, the body is in full compensation. **(M-S)**

▶ The Tensilon (edrophonium) test is used to confirm myasthenia gravis. **(M-S)**

▶ A masklike facial expression is a sign of myasthenia gravis and Parkinson's disease. **(M-S)**

▶ A sign of Paget's disease is bowleggedness. **(M-S)**

▶ For the patient abiding by Jewish custom, milk and meat shouldn't be served in the same meal. **(FND)**

▶ Hyperalertness and the startle reflex are characteristics of post-traumatic stress disorder. **(PSY)**

▶ A treatment for a phobia is desensitization, a process in which the patient is slowly exposed to the stimuli about which the phobia exists. **(PSY)**

▶ Albumin is a colloid that aids in maintaining fluid within the vascular system. If albumin were filtered out through the kidneys into the urine, edema in the body would occur. **(M-S)**

▶ Edema from water and trauma won't pit. **(M-S)**

▶ Dehydration is water loss only; fluid volume deficit refers to all fluids in the body. **(M-S)**

▶ To maintain fluid balance, normal saline solution should be used when giving an enema to an infant. **(PED)**

▶ The primary action of an oil retention enema is to lubricate the colon with a secondary action of softening the stools. **(M-S)**

▶ Glucose in the urine in the early stages of pregnancy may be related to the increased shunting of glucose to the developing placenta without a corresponding increased reabsorption capability of the kidneys. **(MAT)**

▶ The patient using a walker should be instructed to move the walker approximately 12″ (30.5 cm) to the front and then advance into the walker. **(M-S)**

▶ Bradykinesia is a sign of Parkinson's disease. **(PED)**

▶ A backward arching curvature of the spine is termed lordosis.
(M-S)

▶ A forward curvature of the spine is termed kyphosis.   **(M-S)**

▶ A common complaint of acute lymphocytic leukemia in the toddler and preschooler is leg pain.   **(PED)**

▶ A positive response to therapy of an individual with anorexia nervosa is sustained weight gain.   **(M-S)**

▶ The medication in dialysate is heparin.   **(M-S)**

▶ A graft removed from one area of the body for transplanting to another is termed autograft.   **(M-S)**

▶ Signs of cervical cancer include midmenses bleeding and post-coital bleeding.   **(M-S)**

▶ The purpose of catheter insertion after a prostatectomy is to irrigate the bladder to keep urine straw-colored or a light pink, to put direct pressure on the operative side, and to maintain a patent urethra.   **(M-S)**

▶ If a radiation implant becomes dislodged but remains in the patient, the nurse should notify the doctor.   **(M-S)**

▶ The best method to reduce the risk for atelectasis is to ambulate the patient.   **(M-S)**

▶ Atelectasis usually occurs 24 to 48 hours after surgery.   **(M-S)**

▶ Patients at the greatest risk for atelectasis are those who have had high abdominal surgery such as cholecystectomy.   **(M-S)**

▶ Persistent decrease in oxygen to the kidneys will result in erythropoiesis.   **(M-S)**

▶ Rhonchi and crackles indicate an ineffective airway clearance in the patient.   **(M-S)**

▶ Wheezing indicates bronchospasms.   **(M-S)**

▶ Clinical signs and symptoms of hypoxemia are restlessness (usually the first sign), agitation, dyspnea, and disorientation.
(M-S)

▶ Common adverse effects of opioids are constipation and respiratory depression.
(M-S)

▶ Disuse osteoporosis is the result of demineralization of calcium secondary to prolonged bed rest.
(M-S)

▶ The best way to prevent disuse osteoporosis is to ambulate the patient.
(M-S)

▶ The patient with premature rupture of the membranes is at great risk for infection if labor doesn't begin within 24 hours.
(MAT)

▶ A cane should be carried on the unaffected side and advanced with the affected extremity.
(M-S)

▶ Steroids shouldn't be used with chickenpox or shingles due to the adverse effect of the drug.
(M-S)

▶ A person seroconverts approximately 3 to 6 months after exposure to human immunodeficiency virus.
(M-S)

▶ The antiviral therapy zidovudine (AZT) is started when the CD4+ T-cell count is 500 cells/µl or less.
(M-S)

▶ Kaposi sarcoma on the light-skinned person will present as a purplish color and as dark brown to black on a dark-skinned person.
(M-S)

▶ After the esophageal balloon tamponade is in place, inflate it to 20 mm Hg.
(M-S)

▶ The patient with Kaposi sarcoma should avoid acidic or highly seasoned foods.
(M-S)

▶ The treatment for oral candidiasis is amphotericin B (Fungizone) or fluconazole (Diflucan).
(M-S)

▶ A sign of respiratory failure is vital capacity less than 15 ml/kg and respiratory rate greater than 30 breaths/minute or less than 8 breaths/minute.
(M-S)

► For left-sided cardiac catheterization, the catheter is threaded through the descending aorta, aortic arch, ascending aorta, aortic valve, and left ventricle. **(M-S)**

► For right-sided cardiac catheterization, the catheter is threaded through the superior vena cava, right atrium, right ventricle, pulmonary artery, and pulmonary capillaries. **(M-S)**

► Anemia can be divided into four groups according to cause: blood loss, impaired production of red blood cells (RBCs), increased destruction of RBCs, and nutritional deficiencies. **(M-S)**

► Aspirin, ibuprofen, phenobarbital, lithium, colchicine, lead, and chloramphenicol are known to cause aplastic anemia. **(M-S)**

► After the patient has a bone marrow aspiration, the nurse should apply direct pressure to the site for 3 to 5 minutes to reduce the risk of bleeding. **(M-S)**

► Fresh frozen plasma is thawed to 98.6° F (37° C) before infusion. **(M-S)**

► Signs of thrombocytopenia include petechiae, ecchymoses, hematuria, and gingival bleeding. **(M-S)**

► The patient with thrombocytopenia should be taught to use a soft toothbrush, avoid rectal instrumentation, and use an electric razor. **(M-S)**

► Signs of fluid overload include increased central venous pressure, increased pulse rate, distended jugular veins, and bounding pulse. **(M-S)**

► The patient with leukopenia (or any other patient at an increased risk for acquiring an infection) should avoid eating raw meats, fresh fruits, and vegetables. **(M-S)**

► The peak age for acute lymphocytic leukemia is ages 2 to 4; the disease usually presents with complaint of pain in the lower extremities. **(PED)**

► The patient undergoing therapy for acute lymphocytic leukemia should have his urine and stools checked for blood. **(PED)**

▶ To prevent a severe graft-versus-host reaction, most commonly seen in patients over age 30, the donor marrow is treated with monoclonal antibodies before transplantation.   **(M-S)**

▶ The four most common signs of hypoglycemia reported by patients are nervousness, mental disorientation, weakness, and perspiration.   **(M-S)**

▶ Prolonged attacks of hypoglycemia in the diabetic patient can result in brain damage.   **(M-S)**

▶ Whether the patient can perform a procedure (psychomotor domain of learning) is a better indicator of the effectiveness of patient teaching than whether the patient can simply state the steps of the procedure (cognitive domain of learning).   **(FND)**

▶ Activities that increase intracranial pressure include coughing, sneezing, straining to pass stools, bending over, and blowing the nose.   **(M-S)**

▶ Treatment for bleeding esophageal varices includes vasopressin, esophageal tamponade, iced saline lavage, and vitamin K.   **(M-S)**

▶ Hepatitis C (also known as blood-transfusion hepatitis) is a parenterally transmitted form of hepatitis with a high incident of carrier status.   **(M-S)**

▶ The nurse should be concerned about fluid and electrolyte problems in the patient who has ascites, edema, decreased urine output, and low blood pressure.   **(M-S)**

▶ The nurse should be concerned about GI bleeding, low blood pressure, and increased heart rate in the patient who is hemorrhaging.   **(M-S)**

▶ The nurse should be concerned about generalized malaise, cloudiness of urine, purulent drainage, tachycardia, and increased temperature in a patient who has an infection.   **(M-S)**

▶ The patient with edema or ascites should have his serum electrolyte level monitored, be weighed daily, have abdominal girth measured with a centimeter tape at same location using the umbilicus as checkpoint, have intake and output measured, and have blood pressure taken at least every 4 hours.   **(M-S)**

▶ Endogenous sources of ammonia include azotemia, GI bleeding, catabolism, and constipation.   **(M-S)**

▶ Exogenous sources of ammonia include protein, blood transfusion, and amino acids.   **(M-S)**

▶ A histologic grading system used to classify cancers is grade 1 (well-differentiated), grade 2 (moderately well-differentiated), grade 3 (poorly differentiated), and grade 4 (very poorly differentiated).   **(M-S)**

▶ A grading system used to classify tumors is T0 (no evidence of a primary tumor; TIS (tumor in situ); and T1, T2, T3, and T4 (according to size and involvement of tumor; the higher the number, the greater the involvement).   **(M-S)**

▶ Symptoms of major depressive disorder include depressed mood, inability to experience pleasure, sleep disturbance, appetite changes, decreased libido, and feelings of worthlessness.   **(PSY)**

▶ Developmental stages according to Erik Erikson are trust versus mistrust (birth to 18 months), autonomy versus shame and doubt (18 months to 3 years), initiative versus guilt (3 to 5 years), industry versus inferiority (5 to 12 years), identity versus identity diffusion (12 to 18 years), intimacy versus isolation (18 to 25 years), generativity versus stagnation (25 to 60 years), and ego integrity versus despair (older than 60 years).   **(FND)**

▶ Psychosexual stages of development according to Sigmund Freud are oral stage (infancy: birth to 1 year), anal stage (toddler: 1 to 3 years), phallic stage (preschool: 3 to 6 years), latency stage (school age: 6 to 12 years), and genital stage (adolescence and young adult: 12 to 18 years).   **(PED)**

▶ Pheochromocytoma is a catecholamine-secreting neoplasm of the adrenal medulla resulting in an excessive production of epinephrine and norepinephrine.   **(M-S)**

▶ Clinical manifestation of pheochromocytoma includes visual disturbance, headaches, hypertension, and elevated serum blood glucose level. **(M-S)**

▶ The patient shouldn't consume any caffeine-containing products, such as cola, coffee, or tea, for at least 8 hours prior to obtaining a 24-hour urine sample for vanillylmandelic acid. **(M-S)**

▶ The patient taking ColBENEMID (probenecid and colchicine) for gout should increase fluid intake to 2,000 ml/day. **(M-S)**

▶ The purpose of administering a miotic such as pilocarpine to the patient with glaucoma is to increase the outflow of aqueous humor, which decreases intraocular tension. **(M-S)**

▶ The drug most used to treat streptococcal pharyngitis and rheumatic fever is penicillin. **(M-S)**

▶ Face the hearing impaired patient when communicating with him. **(FND)**

▶ The patient with gout should avoid purine-containing foods, such as liver and other organ meats. **(M-S)**

▶ The patient undergoing magnetic resonance imaging will lie on a flat platform, which moves through a magnetic field. **(M-S)**

▶ Infants of diabetic mothers are prone to macrosomia related to increased insulin production in the fetus. **(MAT)**

▶ Laboratory values in bacterial meningitis include increased white blood cell count, increased protein, increased lactic acid, and decreased glucose level. **(M-S)**

▶ To promote rest for the young child with meningitis, decrease environmental stimulation. **(PED)**

▶ Mannitol is a hypertonic osmotic diuretic, which decreases intracranial pressure. **(M-S)**

▶ The best method to debride a wound is to use a wet-to-dry dressing and remove the dressing when it has dried. **(M-S)**

▶ Patients who have had chest wall injuries, chest wall surgeries, and surgery in the upper abdomen are at the greatest risk for developing respiratory complications.   **(M-S)**

▶ Secondary methods for preventing postoperative respiratory complications include having the patient use an incentive spirometer, turning the patient, advising the patient to cough and deep breath, and hydrating the patient.   **(M-S)**

▶ The nurse shouldn't put anything (including a thermometer) in the mouth of the child who is suspected of having epiglottitis.   **(PED)**

▶ To prevent heat loss in the newborn, bathe one part of his body at a time and keep the rest of the body covered.   **(MAT)**

▶ A characteristic of allergic inspiratory and expiratory wheezing is a dry, hacking, nonproductive cough.   **(M-S)**

▶ The incubation period for Rocky Mountain spotted fever ranges from 7 to 14 days.   **(M-S)**

▶ A spiral fracture of the humerus in the child may indicate child abuse.   **(PED)**

▶ Miconazole (Monistat) vaginal suppository should be administered with the patient lying flat.   **(M-S)**

▶ The nurse should place the patient who is having a seizure on his side.   **(M-S)**

▶ Signs of hip dislocation are one limb shorter than the other and one limb externally rotated.   **(M-S)**

▶ The purpose of administering anticholinergic medication to the patient before surgery is to diminish secretion of saliva and gastric juices.   **(M-S)**

▶ Extrapyramidal syndrome seen in the patient with Parkinson's disease is most likely caused by a deficiency of dopamine in the substantia nigra of the brain.   **(M-S)**

▶ Order of concern in a burn patient is airway, circulation, pain, and infection.   **(M-S)**

▶ A proper nursing intervention for the spouse of the patient who has suffered a serious incapacitating disease is to assist him in mobilizing a support system. **(FND)**

▶ Hyperkalemia normally occurs during the hypovolemic phase in the patient who has sustained a serious burn. **(M-S)**

▶ Black stools in the burn patient are most likely related to a Curling's ulcer. **(M-S)**

▶ Immediate care of a full-thickness skin graft in the patient with burns includes covering the site with a bulky dressing. **(M-S)**

▶ The donor site of a skin graft should be left exposed to the air. **(M-S)**

▶ Any leaking around the T tube should be reported immediately to the doctor. **(M-S)**

▶ The patient who has a cesarean section is at greater risk for developing an infection than the patient who gives birth vaginally. **(MAT)**

▶ The patient with Ménière's disease should be maintained on a low-sodium diet. **(M-S)**

▶ In caring for any postoperative patient, the priority of concern is airway, breathing, circulation, followed by self-care deficits. **(M-S)**

▶ Symptoms associated with myasthenia gravis are most likely related to nerve degeneration. **(M-S)**

▶ Symptoms of septic shock include cold clammy skin, hypotension, and decreased urine output. **(M-S)**

▶ Ninety-five percent of the women with gonorrhea are asymptomatic. **(M-S)**

▶ A sign of tinea capitis in the child is a scratch on the scalp. **(PED)**

▶ Permethrin (Nix) shampoo for head lice has been effective if there are no lice in the hair and no eggs (nits) fixed to hair shafts. **(PED)**

▶ An adverse sign in the patient with a Steinmann's pin in the femur would be erythema, edema, and pain around the pin site. **(M-S)**

▶ Signs of chronic glaucoma include halos around lights, gradual loss of peripheral vision, and cloudiness of vision. **(M-S)**

▶ Signs of a detached retina include a sensation of a veil (or curtain) in the line of sight. **(M-S)**

▶ Toxic levels of streptomycin can cause hearing loss. **(M-S)**

▶ A long-term effect of rheumatic fever is mitral valve damage. **(M-S)**

▶ Laboratory values noted in rheumatic fever include an antistreptolysin-O titer, presence of C-reactive protein, leukocytosis, and increased erythrocyte sedimentation rate. **(M-S)**

▶ Crampy pain in the right lower quadrant of the abdomen is a consistent finding in Crohn's disease. **(M-S)**

▶ Crampy pain in the left lower quadrant of the abdomen is a consistent finding in diverticulitis. **(M-S)**

▶ In the icteric phase of hepatitis, urine is amber, stools are clay-colored, and the skin is yellow. **(M-S)**

▶ The occurrence of thrush in the neonate is probably caused by contact with the organism during delivery through the birth canal. **(MAT)**

▶ Signs of osteomyelitis include pathological fractures, shortening or lengthening of the bone, and pain deep in the bone. **(M-S)**

▶ The laboratory test that would best reflect fluid loss because of a burn would be the hematocrit. **(M-S)**

▶ Before administering digoxin to the infant, a nurse should take the apical pulse for 1 full minute. **(PED)**

▶ To determine how much urine is in a diaper, the nurse should weigh the wet diaper, subtract the weight of a dry diaper, and convert each gram to a milliliter. **(PED)**

▶ The patient experiencing acute pancreatitis should take nothing by mouth and have gastric suction to decompress the stomach. **(M-S)**

▶ The purpose of a mist tent is to increase the hydration of secretions. **(M-S)**

▶ The level of mist in a tent should never be so thick as to impede the viewing of the patient's breathing pattern. **(M-S)**

▶ The patient on levodopa should avoid foods that contain pyridoxine (vitamin B_6), such as beans, tuna, and beef liver, because it decreases the effectiveness of levodopa. **(M-S)**

▶ The patient with a transactional injury of C3 will need positive ventilation. **(M-S)**

▶ The action of phenytoin (Dilantin) is potentiated when given with anticoagulants. **(M-S)**

▶ Cerebral palsy is a nonprogressive disorder that persists throughout life. **(M-S)**

▶ The nurse should keep the sac of meningomyelocele moist with normal saline solution. **(MAT)**

▶ A consistent finding in the child with meningococcal meningitis is purpuric skin rash. **(PED)**

▶ The treatment for the conscious toddler who has swallowed liquid drain cleaner is dilute vinegar solution. **(PED)**

▶ A complication of ulcerative colitis is perforation. **(M-S)**

▶ For the patient with multiple sclerosis experiencing diplopia, patch one eye. **(M-S)**

▶ A danger sign following a hip replacement is a lack of reflexes in the affected extremity. **(M-S)**

▶ A clinical manifestation of a ruptured lumbar disk includes pain shooting down the leg and terminating in the popliteal space. **(M-S)**

▶ For the baby in a body cast, tuck a diaper in the perineal area to prevent urine from flowing back into the cast. **(PED)**

▶ The most important nutritional need of the burn patient is I.V. fluid with electrolytes. **(M-S)**

▶ Have the child bend over toward his knees after he has been administered syrup of ipecac. **(PED)**

▶ The patient with systemic lupus erythematosus should avoid sunshine, hair spray, hair color, and dusting powder. **(M-S)**

▶ Poor hygiene is a contributing factor to the development of impetigo. **(PED)**

▶ The best position for the patient with low back pain is sitting in a straight-backed chair. **(M-S)**

▶ Clinical signs of ulcerative colitis include bloody, purulent, mucoid, and watery stools. **(M-S)**

▶ The patient with a protein systemic shunt needs a lifelong protein-restricted diet. **(M-S)**

▶ The patient with a hiatal hernia should maintain an upright position after eating. **(M-S)**

▶ Keep a suction apparatus at the bedside of the patient at risk for status epilepticus. **(M-S)**

▶ The leading cause of death in the burn patient is respiratory compromise. **(M-S)**

▶ Signs of scoliosis include limping walk, uneven hemline, and asymmetrical breast. **(PED)**

▶ A measles-mumps-rubella vaccine shouldn't be given before age 12 months. **(PED)**

▶ An early sign of lead poisoning is drowsiness. **(PED)**

▶ Late signs of lead poisoning are seizures and irreversible brain damage. **(PED)**

▶ Pertussis vaccine shouldn't be given to the child with blood positive for human immunodeficiency virus antibodies. **(PED)**

▶ The priority concern for the patient with herpes zoster is pain management. **(M-S)**

▶ The treatment for Rocky Mountain spotted fever is tetracycline. **(M-S)**

▶ Strawberry tongue is a sign of scarlet fever. **(M-S)**

▶ Parents should inspect the bed linen of the child who has myringotomy tubes daily to make sure that the tubes haven't fallen out. **(PED)**

▶ If the patient is suffering from hemianopia, the nurse should place the call light, the meal tray, and other items in his field of vision. **(M-S)**

▶ The toddler in a crib should have a crib net. **(PED)**

▶ The child shouldn't be asked a "yes" or "no" question unless the nurse plans on going along with the child's wishes. **(PED)**

▶ A sign of Paget's disease are bow legs. **(PED)**

▶ The purpose of Buck's traction is to reduce muscle spasms. **(PED)**

▶ The best position for the patient following a craniotomy is semi-Fowler's. **(M-S)**

▶ The parent of the child with a cast should watch for edema, which causes decreased capillary refill. **(PED)**

▶ Signs of renal trauma include flank pain, hematoma and, possibly, decreased urine output. **(M-S)**

▶ Flank pain and hematoma in the back indicate renal hemorrhage in the trauma patient. **(M-S)**

▶ Natural diuretics include coffee, tea, and grapefruit juice. **(M-S)**

▶ Central venous pressure of 18 cm H_2O indicates hypervolemia.
(M-S)

▶ Clinical signs of lithium toxicity are nausea, vomiting, and lethargy. **(PSY)**

▶ Salmonellosis can be acquired by eating contaminated meats and eggs. **(M-S)**

▶ Good sources of magnesium include fish, nuts, and grains.
(M-S)

▶ Patients with low blood urea nitrogen levels should be instructed to eat high-protein foods, such as fish and chicken.
(M-S)

▶ The nurse should monitor the patient with Guillain-Barré syndrome for respiratory compromise. **(M-S)**

▶ A heating pad may provide comfort to the patient with pelvic inflammatory disease. **(M-S)**

▶ After the patient has supratentorial surgery, the nurse should place the patient in a semi-Fowler position. **(M-S)**

▶ To prevent deep vein thrombosis, have the patient exercise legs at least every 2 hours, elevate the patient's legs above the level of the heart while lying down, and help the patient ambulate.
(M-S)

▶ Following a bronchoscopy procedure, check the patient's gag reflex. **(M-S)**

▶ Abdominal pain and pain that radiates to the left shoulder may indicate a ruptured spleen in the patient with mononucleosis.
(M-S)

▶ For a skin graft to take, it must be autologous. **(M-S)**

▶ Untreated retinal detachment will lead to blindness. **(M-S)**

▶ The diet for the patient with fibrocystic breast disease should be low in caffeine and salt. **(M-S)**

▶ A foul odor at the pin site of the patient in skeletal traction would indicate infection. **(M-S)**

▶ A muscle relaxant administered with oxygen may cause malignant hyperthermia and respiratory depression. **(M-S)**

▶ Pain on movement of the cervix, together with adnexal tenderness, may suggest pelvic inflammatory disease. **(M-S)**

▶ Asking too many "why" questions yields scant information and may overwhelm the psychiatric patient, which can lead to stress and withdrawal. **(PSY)**

▶ Fundal height that falls short of expectations by more than 2 cm may be due to growth retardation, missed abortion, transverse lie, or false pregnancy. **(MAT)**

▶ In cyanotic congenital heart defects, unoxygenated blood is shunted from the right side of the heart to the left, where it flows through the left ventricle to all parts of the body, resulting in cyanosis. **(PED)**

▶ Fundal height that exceeds expectations by more than 2 cm may be due to multiple gestation, polyhydramnios, uterine myomata, or a big baby. **(MAT)**

▶ Remote memory may be impaired in late stages of dementia. **(PSY)**

▶ Tetralogy of Fallot consists of four separate defects — ventricular septal defect, overriding aorta, pulmonary stenosis, and right ventricular hypertrophy. **(PED)**

▶ Crisis intervention aims to restore the person to a precrisis level of functioning and order. **(M-S)**

▶ According to the *DSM-IV*, a bipolar II disorder is characterized by at least one manic episode accompanied by hypomania. **(PSY)**

▶ Congenital heart defects are classified as cyanotic or acyanotic. **(PED)**

▶ Nephrotic syndrome is marked by proteinuria, hypoalbuminemia, and edema and sometimes hematuria, hypertension, and a decreased glomerular filtration rate.   **(M-S)**

▶ Acute glomerulonephritis, the most common noninfectious renal disease of childhood, is usually caused by a reaction to streptococcal infection.   **(PED)**

▶ Hydrocephalus may be congenital or may result from a tumor, infection, or hemorrhage.   **(PED)**

▶ Hyperpyrexia refers to extreme elevation in temperature above 106° F (41.1° C).   **(FND)**

▶ Bowel sounds may be heard over a hernia but not over a hydrocele.   **(M-S)**

▶ S_1 is decreased in first-degree heart block, and S_2 is decreased in aortic stenosis.   **(M-S)**

▶ Gas in the colon may produce tympany in the right upper quadrant, obscure liver dullness, and lead to falsely decreased estimates of liver size.   **(M-S)**

▶ In ataxia due to loss of position sense, vision compensates for the sensory loss and the patient stands fairly well with eyes open but loses balance when they're closed, indicating a positive Romberg test.   **(M-S)**

▶ The patient's inability to recognize numbers when drawn on the hand with the blunt end of a pen suggests a lesion in the sensory cortex.   **(M-S)**

▶ Dilated scalp veins indicate long-standing increased intracranial pressure.   **(PED)**

Index